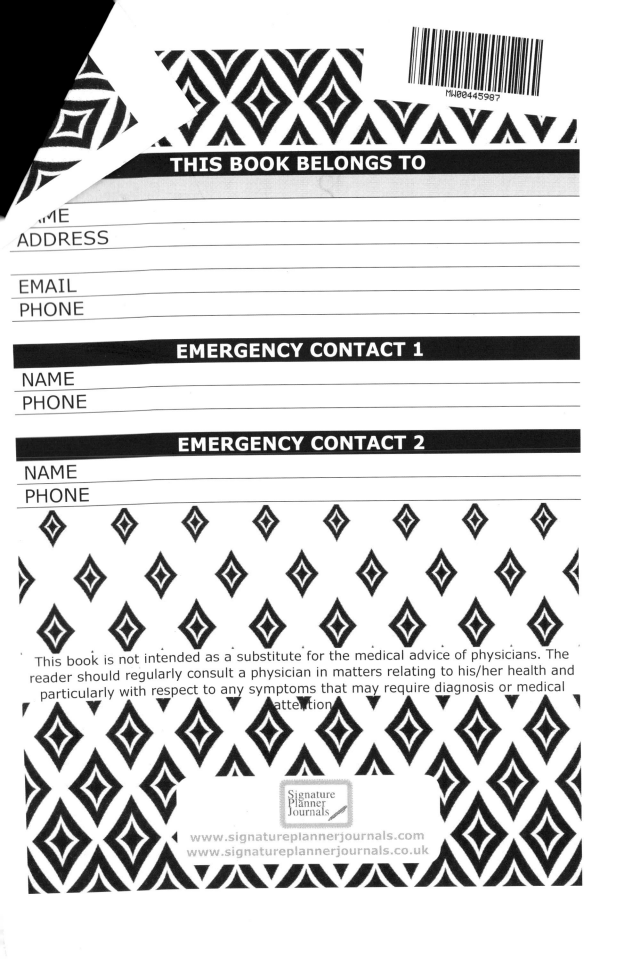

MW00445987

THIS BOOK BELONGS TO

NAME

ADDRESS

EMAIL

PHONE

EMERGENCY CONTACT 1

NAME

PHONE

EMERGENCY CONTACT 2

NAME

PHONE

This book is not intended as a substitute for the medical advice of physicians. The reader should regularly consult a physician in matters relating to his/her health and particularly with respect to any symptoms that may require diagnosis or medical attention.

Signature Planner Journals

www.signatureplannerjournals.com
www.signatureplannerjournals.co.uk

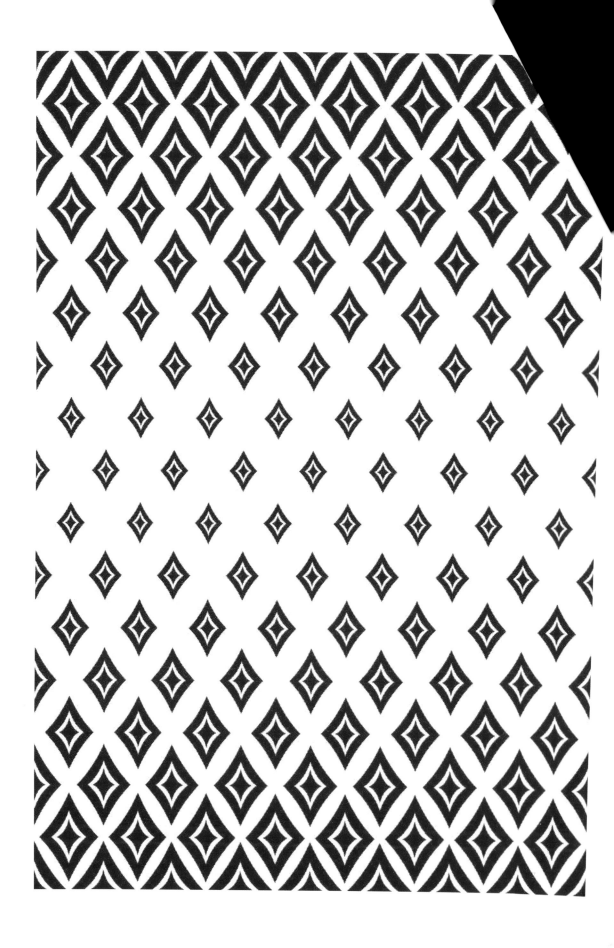

CONTENTS

❖ Chronic Pain Assessment Pages 1

❖ Treatment History- Prescription Medication 101

❖ Doctors/ Clinic Appointments 105

❖ Notes 111

CHRONIC PAIN ASSESSMENT

DATE		DAY	
TIME STARTED		TIME ENDED	
TOTAL DURATION			

RIGHT SIDE   BACK   FRONT   LEFT SIDE

LEFT RIGHT   RIGHT LEFT

←   Mark the location of the pain

LENGTH OF TIME EXPERIENCING THE PAIN?

< 6 Months		6-12 Months	
1-3 Years		3 Years +	

TYPE OF PAIN

Indescribable		Stabbing		Sharp	
Burning		Aching		Prickly	
Numb		Tingling/ Pins & Needles			
Other					

EXTERNAL ENVIROMENTAL FACTORS

Sun/ Heat		Cold		Windy	
Rain		Aching		Cloudy	
Other					

PAIN SCALE

NO PAIN   ————————————————————→   SEVERE PAIN

0	1	2	3	4	5	6	7	8	9	10

SUSPECTED TRIGGERS

-          •
-          •
-          •
-          •

SYMPTOMS

RELIEF MEASURES

NOTES

CHRONIC PAIN ASSESSMENT

DATE		DAY	
TIME STARTED		TIME ENDED	
TOTAL DURATION			

RIGHT SIDE   BACK   FRONT   LEFT SIDE

LEFT   RIGHT   RIGHT   LEFT

Mark the location of the pain

LENGTH OF TIME EXPERIENCING THE PAIN?

< 6 Months		6-12 Months	
1-3 Years		3 Years +	

TYPE OF PAIN

Indescribable		Stabbing		Sharp	
Burning		Aching		Prickly	
Numb		Tingling/ Pins & Needles			
Other					

EXTERNAL ENVIROMENTAL FACTORS

Sun/ Heat		Cold		Windy	
Rain		Aching		Cloudy	
Other					

PAIN SCALE

NO PAIN ⟶ SEVERE PAIN

0	1	2	3	4	5	6	7	8	9	10

SUSPECTED TRIGGERS

-
-
-
-

-
-
-
-

SYMPTOMS

RELIEF MEASURES

NOTES

CHRONIC PAIN ASSESSMENT

DATE		DAY	
TIME STARTED		TIME ENDED	
TOTAL DURATION			

RIGHT SIDE   BACK   FRONT   LEFT SIDE

LEFT   RIGHT   RIGHT   LEFT

←   Mark the location of the pain

LENGTH OF TIME EXPERIENCING THE PAIN?

< 6 Months			6-12 Months	
1-3 Years			3 Years +	

TYPE OF PAIN

Indescribable		Stabbing		Sharp	
Burning		Aching		Prickly	
Numb		Tingling/ Pins & Needles			
Other					

EXTERNAL ENVIROMENTAL FACTORS

Sun/ Heat		Cold		Windy	
Rain		Aching		Cloudy	
Other					

PAIN SCALE

NO PAIN   ————————————————→   SEVERE PAIN

0	1	2	3	4	5	6	7	8	9	10

SUSPECTED TRIGGERS

-
-
-
-

-
-
-
-

SYMPTOMS

RELIEF MEASURES

NOTES

CHRONIC PAIN ASSESSMENT

DATE		DAY	
TIME STARTED		**TIME ENDED**	
TOTAL DURATION			

RIGHT SIDE   BACK   FRONT   LEFT SIDE

LEFT   RIGHT   RIGHT   LEFT

←   Mark the location of the pain

LENGTH OF TIME EXPERIENCING THE PAIN?

< 6 Months		6-12 Months	
1-3 Years		3 Years +	

TYPE OF PAIN

Indescribable		Stabbing		Sharp	
Burning		Aching		Prickly	
Numb		Tingling/ Pins & Needles			
Other					

EXTERNAL ENVIROMENTAL FACTORS

Sun/ Heat		Cold		Windy	
Rain		Aching		Cloudy	
Other					

PAIN SCALE

NO PAIN ————————————————→ SEVERE PAIN

0	1	2	3	4	5	6	7	8	9	10

SUSPECTED TRIGGERS

-
-
-
-

-
-
-
-

SYMPTOMS

RELIEF MEASURES

NOTES

CHRONIC PAIN ASSESSMENT

DATE		DAY	
TIME STARTED		TIME ENDED	
TOTAL DURATION			

RIGHT SIDE   BACK   FRONT   LEFT SIDE

LEFT RIGHT   RIGHT LEFT

← Mark the location of the pain

LENGTH OF TIME EXPERIENCING THE PAIN?

< 6 Months		6-12 Months	
1-3 Years		3 Years +	

TYPE OF PAIN

Indescribable		Stabbing		Sharp	
Burning		Aching		Prickly	
Numb		Tingling/ Pins & Needles			
Other					

EXTERNAL ENVIROMENTAL FACTORS

Sun/ Heat		Cold		Windy	
Rain		Aching		Cloudy	
Other					

PAIN SCALE

NO PAIN ⟶ SEVERE PAIN

0	1	2	3	4	5	6	7	8	9	10

SUSPECTED TRIGGERS

-
-
-
-

-
-
-
-

SYMPTOMS

RELIEF MEASURES

NOTES

DATE		DAY	
TIME STARTED		TIME ENDED	
TOTAL DURATION			

RIGHT SIDE   BACK   FRONT   LEFT SIDE

LEFT RIGHT   RIGHT LEFT

← ────── Mark the location of the pain

LENGTH OF TIME EXPERIENCING THE PAIN?

< 6 Months		6-12 Months	
1-3 Years		3 Years +	

TYPE OF PAIN

Indescribable		Stabbing		Sharp	
Burning		Aching		Prickly	
Numb		Tingling/ Pins & Needles			
Other					

EXTERNAL ENVIROMENTAL FACTORS

Sun/ Heat		Cold		Windy	
Rain		Aching		Cloudy	
Other					

PAIN SCALE

NO PAIN ─────────────────────→ SEVERE PAIN

0	1	2	3	4	5	6	7	8	9	10

SUSPECTED TRIGGERS

-
-
-
-

-
-
-
-

SYMPTOMS

RELIEF MEASURES

NOTES

CHRONIC PAIN ASSESSMENT

DATE		DAY	
TIME STARTED		TIME ENDED	
TOTAL DURATION			

RIGHT SIDE   BACK   FRONT   LEFT SIDE

← Mark the location of the pain

LENGTH OF TIME EXPERIENCING THE PAIN?

< 6 Months		6-12 Months	
1-3 Years		3 Years +	

TYPE OF PAIN

Indescribable		Stabbing		Sharp	
Burning		Aching		Prickly	
Numb		Tingling/ Pins & Needles			
Other					

EXTERNAL ENVIROMENTAL FACTORS

Sun/ Heat		Cold		Windy	
Rain		Aching		Cloudy	
Other					

PAIN SCALE

NO PAIN ——————————————→ SEVERE PAIN

0	1	2	3	4	5	6	7	8	9	10

SUSPECTED TRIGGERS

- _____
- _____
- _____
- _____

- _____
- _____
- _____
- _____

SYMPTOMS

_____
_____
_____
_____
_____
_____
_____
_____

RELIEF MEASURES

_____
_____
_____
_____
_____

NOTES

_____
_____
_____
_____

CHRONIC PAIN ASSESSMENT

DATE		DAY	
TIME STARTED		**TIME ENDED**	
TOTAL DURATION			

RIGHT SIDE   BACK   FRONT   LEFT SIDE

LEFT   RIGHT   RIGHT   LEFT

← Mark the location of the pain

LENGTH OF TIME EXPERIENCING THE PAIN?

< 6 Months		6-12 Months	
1-3 Years		3 Years +	

TYPE OF PAIN

Indescribable		Stabbing		Sharp	
Burning		Aching		Prickly	
Numb		Tingling/ Pins & Needles			
Other					

EXTERNAL ENVIROMENTAL FACTORS

Sun/ Heat		Cold		Windy	
Rain		Aching		Cloudy	
Other					

PAIN SCALE

NO PAIN ——————————————————→ SEVERE PAIN

0	1	2	3	4	5	6	7	8	9	10

SUSPECTED TRIGGERS

-
-
-
-

-
-
-
-

SYMPTOMS

RELIEF MEASURES

NOTES

CHRONIC PAIN ASSESSMENT

DATE		DAY	
TIME STARTED		TIME ENDED	
TOTAL DURATION			

RIGHT SIDE   BACK   FRONT   LEFT SIDE

LEFT   RIGHT   RIGHT   LEFT

←   Mark the location of the pain

LENGTH OF TIME EXPERIENCING THE PAIN?

< 6 Months			6-12 Months	
1-3 Years			3 Years +	

TYPE OF PAIN

Indescribable		Stabbing		Sharp	
Burning		Aching		Prickly	
Numb		Tingling/ Pins & Needles			
Other					

EXTERNAL ENVIROMENTAL FACTORS

Sun/ Heat		Cold		Windy	
Rain		Aching		Cloudy	
Other					

PAIN SCALE

NO PAIN ——————————————————→ SEVERE PAIN

0	1	2	3	4	5	6	7	8	9	10

SUSPECTED TRIGGERS

-      •
-      •
-      •
-      •

SYMPTOMS

RELIEF MEASURES

NOTES

CHRONIC PAIN ASSESSMENT

DATE		DAY		
TIME STARTED		TIME ENDED		
TOTAL DURATION				

RIGHT SIDE · BACK · FRONT · LEFT SIDE

LEFT · RIGHT · RIGHT · LEFT

← Mark the location of the pain

LENGTH OF TIME EXPERIENCING THE PAIN?

< 6 Months		6-12 Months
1-3 Years		3 Years +

TYPE OF PAIN

Indescribable	Stabbing		Sharp
Burning	Aching		Prickly
Numb	Tingling/ Pins & Needles		
Other			

EXTERNAL ENVIROMENTAL FACTORS

Sun/ Heat		Cold	Windy
Rain		Aching	Cloudy
Other			

PAIN SCALE

NO PAIN → SEVERE PAIN

0	1	2	3	4	5	6	7	8	9	10

SUSPECTED TRIGGERS

-
-
-
-

-
-
-
-

SYMPTOMS

RELIEF MEASURES

NOTES

CHRONIC PAIN ASSESSMENT

DATE		DAY	
TIME STARTED		TIME ENDED	
TOTAL DURATION			

RIGHT SIDE   BACK   FRONT   LEFT SIDE

LEFT   RIGHT   RIGHT   LEFT

← Mark the location of the pain

LENGTH OF TIME EXPERIENCING THE PAIN?

< 6 Months		6-12 Months	
1-3 Years		3 Years +	

TYPE OF PAIN

Indescribable		Stabbing		Sharp	
Burning		Aching		Prickly	
Numb		Tingling/ Pins & Needles			
Other					

EXTERNAL ENVIROMENTAL FACTORS

Sun/ Heat		Cold		Windy	
Rain		Aching		Cloudy	
Other					

PAIN SCALE

NO PAIN ────────────────────────→ SEVERE PAIN

0	1	2	3	4	5	6	7	8	9	10

SUSPECTED TRIGGERS

-
-
-
-

-
-
-
-

SYMPTOMS

RELIEF MEASURES

NOTES

CHRONIC PAIN ASSESSMENT

DATE		DAY	
TIME STARTED		TIME ENDED	
TOTAL DURATION			

RIGHT SIDE   BACK   FRONT   LEFT SIDE

LEFT   RIGHT   RIGHT   LEFT

← Mark the location of the pain

LENGTH OF TIME EXPERIENCING THE PAIN?

< 6 Months		6-12 Months
1-3 Years		3 Years +

TYPE OF PAIN

Indescribable	Stabbing		Sharp
Burning	Aching		Prickly
Numb	Tingling/ Pins & Needles		
Other			

EXTERNAL ENVIROMENTAL FACTORS

Sun/ Heat		Cold	Windy
Rain		Aching	Cloudy
Other			

PAIN SCALE

NO PAIN ———————————————→ SEVERE PAIN

0	1	2	3	4	5	6	7	8	9	10

SUSPECTED TRIGGERS

-      •
-      •
-      •
-      •

SYMPTOMS

RELIEF MEASURES

NOTES

CHRONIC PAIN ASSESSMENT

DATE		DAY	
TIME STARTED		TIME ENDED	
TOTAL DURATION			

RIGHT SIDE   BACK   FRONT   LEFT SIDE

LEFT   RIGHT   RIGHT   LEFT

← _____ Mark the location of the pain

LENGTH OF TIME EXPERIENCING THE PAIN?

< 6 Months		6-12 Months	
1-3 Years		3 Years +	

TYPE OF PAIN

Indescribable		Stabbing		Sharp	
Burning		Aching		Prickly	
Numb		Tingling/ Pins & Needles			
Other					

EXTERNAL ENVIROMENTAL FACTORS

Sun/ Heat		Cold		Windy	
Rain		Aching		Cloudy	
Other					

PAIN SCALE

NO PAIN _____→ SEVERE PAIN

0	1	2	3	4	5	6	7	8	9	10

SUSPECTED TRIGGERS

-
-
-
-

-
-
-
-

SYMPTOMS

RELIEF MEASURES

NOTES

CHRONIC PAIN ASSESSMENT

DATE		DAY	
TIME STARTED		TIME ENDED	
TOTAL DURATION			

RIGHT SIDE BACK FRONT LEFT SIDE

LEFT RIGHT RIGHT LEFT

← Mark the location of the pain

LENGTH OF TIME EXPERIENCING THE PAIN?

< 6 Months			6-12 Months
1-3 Years			3 Years +

TYPE OF PAIN

Indescribable		Stabbing		Sharp	
Burning		Aching		Prickly	
Numb		Tingling/ Pins & Needles			
Other					

EXTERNAL ENVIROMENTAL FACTORS

Sun/ Heat		Cold		Windy	
Rain		Aching		Cloudy	
Other					

PAIN SCALE

NO PAIN ——————————————→ SEVERE PAIN

0	1	2	3	4	5	6	7	8	9	10

SUSPECTED TRIGGERS

-
-
-
-

-
-
-
-

SYMPTOMS

RELIEF MEASURES

NOTES

CHRONIC PAIN ASSESSMENT

DATE		DAY	
TIME STARTED		TIME ENDED	
TOTAL DURATION			

RIGHT SIDE BACK FRONT LEFT SIDE

LEFT RIGHT RIGHT LEFT

← Mark the location of the pain

LENGTH OF TIME EXPERIENCING THE PAIN?

< 6 Months		6-12 Months	
1-3 Years		3 Years +	

TYPE OF PAIN

Indescribable		Stabbing		Sharp	
Burning		Aching		Prickly	
Numb		Tingling/ Pins & Needles			
Other					

EXTERNAL ENVIROMENTAL FACTORS

Sun/ Heat		Cold		Windy	
Rain		Aching		Cloudy	
Other					

PAIN SCALE

NO PAIN ————————————————→ SEVERE PAIN

0	1	2	3	4	5	6	7	8	9	10

SUSPECTED TRIGGERS

-
-
-
-

-
-
-
-

SYMPTOMS

RELIEF MEASURES

NOTES

CHRONIC PAIN ASSESSMENT

DATE		DAY	
TIME STARTED		**TIME ENDED**	
TOTAL DURATION			

RIGHT SIDE   BACK   FRONT   LEFT SIDE

LEFT   RIGHT   RIGHT   LEFT

← Mark the location of the pain

LENGTH OF TIME EXPERIENCING THE PAIN?

< 6 Months		6-12 Months	
1-3 Years		3 Years +	

TYPE OF PAIN

Indescribable		Stabbing		Sharp	
Burning		Aching		Prickly	
Numb		Tingling/ Pins & Needles			
Other					

EXTERNAL ENVIROMENTAL FACTORS

Sun/ Heat		Cold		Windy	
Rain		Aching		Cloudy	
Other					

PAIN SCALE

NO PAIN ➡ SEVERE PAIN

0	1	2	3	4	5	6	7	8	9	10

SUSPECTED TRIGGERS

-
-
-
-

-
-
-
-

SYMPTOMS

RELIEF MEASURES

NOTES

CHRONIC PAIN ASSESSMENT

DATE		DAY	
TIME STARTED		TIME ENDED	
TOTAL DURATION			

RIGHT SIDE   BACK   FRONT   LEFT SIDE

LEFT   RIGHT   RIGHT   LEFT

← Mark the location of the pain

LENGTH OF TIME EXPERIENCING THE PAIN?

< 6 Months		6-12 Months	
1-3 Years		3 Years +	

TYPE OF PAIN

Indescribable		Stabbing		Sharp	
Burning		Aching		Prickly	
Numb		Tingling/ Pins & Needles			
Other					

EXTERNAL ENVIROMENTAL FACTORS

Sun/ Heat		Cold		Windy	
Rain		Aching		Cloudy	
Other					

PAIN SCALE

NO PAIN ⟶ SEVERE PAIN

0	1	2	3	4	5	6	7	8	9	10

SUSPECTED TRIGGERS

-
-
-
-

-
-
-
-

SYMPTOMS

RELIEF MEASURES

NOTES

CHRONIC PAIN ASSESSMENT

DATE		DAY	
TIME STARTED		TIME ENDED	
TOTAL DURATION			

RIGHT SIDE   BACK   FRONT   LEFT SIDE

LEFT   RIGHT   RIGHT   LEFT

← Mark the location of the pain

LENGTH OF TIME EXPERIENCING THE PAIN?

< 6 Months		6-12 Months	
1-3 Years		3 Years +	

TYPE OF PAIN

Indescribable		Stabbing		Sharp	
Burning		Aching		Prickly	
Numb		Tingling/ Pins & Needles			
Other					

EXTERNAL ENVIROMENTAL FACTORS

Sun/ Heat		Cold		Windy	
Rain		Aching		Cloudy	
Other					

PAIN SCALE

NO PAIN ———————————————————→ SEVERE PAIN

0	1	2	3	4	5	6	7	8	9	10

SUSPECTED TRIGGERS

-
-
-
-

-
-
-
-

SYMPTOMS

RELIEF MEASURES

NOTES

CHRONIC PAIN ASSESSMENT

DATE		DAY	
TIME STARTED		TIME ENDED	
TOTAL DURATION			

RIGHT SIDE   BACK   FRONT   LEFT SIDE

LEFT   RIGHT   RIGHT   LEFT

← Mark the location of the pain

LENGTH OF TIME EXPERIENCING THE PAIN?

< 6 Months		6-12 Months	
1-3 Years		3 Years +	

TYPE OF PAIN

Indescribable		Stabbing		Sharp	
Burning		Aching		Prickly	
Numb		Tingling/ Pins & Needles			
Other					

EXTERNAL ENVIROMENTAL FACTORS

Sun/ Heat		Cold		Windy	
Rain		Aching		Cloudy	
Other					

PAIN SCALE

NO PAIN ⟶ SEVERE PAIN

0	1	2	3	4	5	6	7	8	9	10

SUSPECTED TRIGGERS

-
-
-
-

-
-
-
-

SYMPTOMS

RELIEF MEASURES

NOTES

DATE		DAY	
TIME STARTED		TIME ENDED	
TOTAL DURATION			

RIGHT SIDE   BACK   FRONT   LEFT SIDE

LEFT RIGHT   RIGHT LEFT

← Mark the location of the pain

LENGTH OF TIME EXPERIENCING THE PAIN?

< 6 Months		6-12 Months	
1-3 Years		3 Years +	

TYPE OF PAIN

Indescribable		Stabbing		Sharp	
Burning		Aching		Prickly	
Numb		Tingling/ Pins & Needles			
Other					

EXTERNAL ENVIROMENTAL FACTORS

Sun/ Heat		Cold		Windy	
Rain		Aching		Cloudy	
Other					

PAIN SCALE

NO PAIN ————————————————→ SEVERE PAIN

0	1	2	3	4	5	6	7	8	9	10

SUSPECTED TRIGGERS

-
-
-
-

-
-
-
-

SYMPTOMS

RELIEF MEASURES

NOTES

CHRONIC PAIN ASSESSMENT

DATE		DAY	
TIME STARTED		TIME ENDED	
TOTAL DURATION			

Mark the location of the pain

LENGTH OF TIME EXPERIENCING THE PAIN?

< 6 Months		6-12 Months
1-3 Years		3 Years +

TYPE OF PAIN

Indescribable		Stabbing		Sharp	
Burning		Aching		Prickly	
Numb		Tingling/ Pins & Needles			
Other					

EXTERNAL ENVIROMENTAL FACTORS

Sun/ Heat		Cold		Windy	
Rain		Aching		Cloudy	
Other					

PAIN SCALE

NO PAIN → SEVERE PAIN

0	1	2	3	4	5	6	7	8	9	10

SUSPECTED TRIGGERS

-
-
-
-

-
-
-
-

SYMPTOMS

RELIEF MEASURES

NOTES

DATE		DAY	
TIME STARTED		TIME ENDED	
TOTAL DURATION			

RIGHT SIDE   BACK   FRONT   LEFT SIDE

LEFT   RIGHT   RIGHT   LEFT

← _____ Mark the location of the pain

LENGTH OF TIME EXPERIENCING THE PAIN?

< 6 Months			6-12 Months
1-3 Years			3 Years +

TYPE OF PAIN

Indescribable		Stabbing		Sharp	
Burning		Aching		Prickly	
Numb		Tingling/ Pins & Needles			
Other					

EXTERNAL ENVIROMENTAL FACTORS

Sun/ Heat			Cold		Windy
Rain			Aching		Cloudy
Other					

PAIN SCALE

NO PAIN _____→ SEVERE PAIN

0	1	2	3	4	5	6	7	8	9	10

SUSPECTED TRIGGERS

- •
- •
- •
- •

- •
- •
- •
- •

SYMPTOMS

RELIEF MEASURES

NOTES

CHRONIC PAIN ASSESSMENT

DATE		DAY	
TIME STARTED		TIME ENDED	
TOTAL DURATION			

RIGHT SIDE   BACK   FRONT   LEFT SIDE

LEFT   RIGHT   RIGHT   LEFT

← ——————— Mark the location of the pain

LENGTH OF TIME EXPERIENCING THE PAIN?

< 6 Months		6-12 Months	
1-3 Years		3 Years +	

TYPE OF PAIN

Indescribable		Stabbing		Sharp	
Burning		Aching		Prickly	
Numb		Tingling/ Pins & Needles			
Other					

EXTERNAL ENVIROMENTAL FACTORS

Sun/ Heat		Cold		Windy	
Rain		Aching		Cloudy	
Other					

PAIN SCALE

NO PAIN ——————————————————→ SEVERE PAIN

0	1	2	3	4	5	6	7	8	9	10

SUSPECTED TRIGGERS

-
-
-
-

-
-
-
-

SYMPTOMS

RELIEF MEASURES

NOTES

CHRONIC PAIN ASSESSMENT

DATE		DAY	
TIME STARTED		**TIME ENDED**	
TOTAL DURATION			

RIGHT SIDE BACK FRONT LEFT SIDE

LEFT RIGHT RIGHT LEFT

← Mark the location of the pain

LENGTH OF TIME EXPERIENCING THE PAIN?

< 6 Months		6-12 Months
1-3 Years		3 Years +

TYPE OF PAIN

Indescribable	Stabbing		Sharp	
Burning	Aching		Prickly	
Numb	Tingling/ Pins & Needles			
Other				

EXTERNAL ENVIROMENTAL FACTORS

Sun/ Heat		Cold		Windy	
Rain		Aching		Cloudy	
Other					

PAIN SCALE

NO PAIN ————————————→ SEVERE PAIN

0	1	2	3	4	5	6	7	8	9	10

SUSPECTED TRIGGERS

-
-
-
-

-
-
-
-

SYMPTOMS

RELIEF MEASURES

NOTES

CHRONIC PAIN ASSESSMENT

DATE		DAY	
TIME STARTED		TIME ENDED	
TOTAL DURATION			

RIGHT SIDE   BACK   FRONT   LEFT SIDE

← Mark the location of the pain

LENGTH OF TIME EXPERIENCING THE PAIN?

< 6 Months			6-12 Months	
1-3 Years			3 Years +	

TYPE OF PAIN

Indescribable		Stabbing		Sharp	
Burning		Aching		Prickly	
Numb		Tingling/ Pins & Needles			
Other					

EXTERNAL ENVIROMENTAL FACTORS

Sun/ Heat		Cold		Windy	
Rain		Aching		Cloudy	
Other					

PAIN SCALE

NO PAIN   ⟶   SEVERE PAIN

0	1	2	3	4	5	6	7	8	9	10

SUSPECTED TRIGGERS

-
-
-
-

-
-
-
-

SYMPTOMS

RELIEF MEASURES

NOTES

CHRONIC PAIN ASSESSMENT

DATE		DAY	
TIME STARTED		**TIME ENDED**	
TOTAL DURATION			

RIGHT SIDE | BACK | FRONT | LEFT SIDE

← Mark the location of the pain

LENGTH OF TIME EXPERIENCING THE PAIN?

< 6 Months		6-12 Months	
1-3 Years		3 Years +	

TYPE OF PAIN

Indescribable		Stabbing		Sharp	
Burning		Aching		Prickly	
Numb		Tingling/ Pins & Needles			
Other					

EXTERNAL ENVIROMENTAL FACTORS

Sun/ Heat		Cold		Windy	
Rain		Aching		Cloudy	
Other					

PAIN SCALE

NO PAIN ——————————→ SEVERE PAIN

0	1	2	3	4	5	6	7	8	9	10

SUSPECTED TRIGGERS

-
-
-
-

-
-
-
-

SYMPTOMS

RELIEF MEASURES

NOTES

CHRONIC PAIN ASSESSMENT

DATE		DAY	
TIME STARTED		TIME ENDED	
TOTAL DURATION			

RIGHT SIDE   BACK   FRONT   LEFT SIDE

LEFT   RIGHT   RIGHT   LEFT

← ———— Mark the location of the pain

LENGTH OF TIME EXPERIENCING THE PAIN?

< 6 Months		6-12 Months	
1-3 Years		3 Years +	

TYPE OF PAIN

Indescribable		Stabbing		Sharp	
Burning		Aching		Prickly	
Numb		Tingling/ Pins & Needles			
Other					

EXTERNAL ENVIROMENTAL FACTORS

Sun/ Heat		Cold		Windy	
Rain		Aching		Cloudy	
Other					

PAIN SCALE

NO PAIN ————————————————→ SEVERE PAIN

0	1	2	3	4	5	6	7	8	9	10

SUSPECTED TRIGGERS

-
-
-
-

-
-
-
-

SYMPTOMS

RELIEF MEASURES

NOTES

CHRONIC PAIN ASSESSMENT

DATE		DAY	
TIME STARTED		**TIME ENDED**	
TOTAL DURATION			

RIGHT SIDE | BACK | FRONT | LEFT SIDE

LEFT | RIGHT | RIGHT | LEFT

← Mark the location of the pain

LENGTH OF TIME EXPERIENCING THE PAIN?

< 6 Months		6-12 Months	
1-3 Years		3 Years +	

TYPE OF PAIN

Indescribable		Stabbing		Sharp	
Burning		Aching		Prickly	
Numb		Tingling/ Pins & Needles			
Other					

EXTERNAL ENVIROMENTAL FACTORS

Sun/ Heat		Cold		Windy	
Rain		Aching		Cloudy	
Other					

PAIN SCALE

NO PAIN →→→ SEVERE PAIN

0	1	2	3	4	5	6	7	8	9	10

SUSPECTED TRIGGERS

-
-
-
-

-
-
-
-

SYMPTOMS

RELIEF MEASURES

NOTES

CHRONIC PAIN ASSESSMENT

DATE		DAY	
TIME STARTED		TIME ENDED	
TOTAL DURATION			

← Mark the location of the pain

LENGTH OF TIME EXPERIENCING THE PAIN?

< 6 Months		6-12 Months	
1-3 Years		3 Years +	

TYPE OF PAIN

Indescribable		Stabbing		Sharp	
Burning		Aching		Prickly	
Numb		Tingling/ Pins & Needles			
Other					

EXTERNAL ENVIROMENTAL FACTORS

Sun/ Heat		Cold		Windy	
Rain		Aching		Cloudy	
Other					

PAIN SCALE

NO PAIN ————————————————→ SEVERE PAIN

0	1	2	3	4	5	6	7	8	9	10

SUSPECTED TRIGGERS

-
-
-
-

-
-
-
-

SYMPTOMS

RELIEF MEASURES

NOTES

CHRONIC PAIN ASSESSMENT

DATE		DAY	
TIME STARTED		TIME ENDED	
TOTAL DURATION			

← Mark the location of the pain

LENGTH OF TIME EXPERIENCING THE PAIN?

< 6 Months		6-12 Months	
1-3 Years		3 Years +	

TYPE OF PAIN

Indescribable	Stabbing		Sharp	
Burning	Aching		Prickly	
Numb	Tingling/ Pins & Needles			
Other				

EXTERNAL ENVIROMENTAL FACTORS

Sun/ Heat		Cold		Windy	
Rain		Aching		Cloudy	
Other					

PAIN SCALE

NO PAIN ─────────────────────→ SEVERE PAIN

0	1	2	3	4	5	6	7	8	9	10

SUSPECTED TRIGGERS

-
-
-
-

-
-
-
-

SYMPTOMS

RELIEF MEASURES

NOTES

CHRONIC PAIN ASSESSMENT

DATE		DAY	
TIME STARTED		TIME ENDED	
TOTAL DURATION			

RIGHT SIDE   BACK   FRONT   LEFT SIDE

LEFT RIGHT   RIGHT LEFT

← Mark the location of the pain

LENGTH OF TIME EXPERIENCING THE PAIN?

< 6 Months		6-12 Months	
1-3 Years		3 Years +	

TYPE OF PAIN

Indescribable		Stabbing		Sharp	
Burning		Aching		Prickly	
Numb		Tingling/ Pins & Needles			
Other					

EXTERNAL ENVIROMENTAL FACTORS

Sun/ Heat		Cold		Windy	
Rain		Aching		Cloudy	
Other					

PAIN SCALE

NO PAIN ————————————————————→ SEVERE PAIN

0	1	2	3	4	5	6	7	8	9	10

SUSPECTED TRIGGERS

-
-
-
-

-
-
-
-

SYMPTOMS

RELIEF MEASURES

NOTES

CHRONIC PAIN ASSESSMENT

DATE		DAY	
TIME STARTED		**TIME ENDED**	
TOTAL DURATION			

RIGHT SIDE   BACK   FRONT   LEFT SIDE

LEFT   RIGHT   RIGHT   LEFT

← ⬅ Mark the location of the pain

LENGTH OF TIME EXPERIENCING THE PAIN?

< 6 Months		6-12 Months	
1-3 Years		3 Years +	

TYPE OF PAIN

Indescribable		Stabbing		Sharp	
Burning		Aching		Prickly	
Numb		Tingling/ Pins & Needles			
Other					

EXTERNAL ENVIROMENTAL FACTORS

Sun/ Heat		Cold		Windy	
Rain		Aching		Cloudy	
Other					

PAIN SCALE

NO PAIN ————————————————→ SEVERE PAIN

0	1	2	3	4	5	6	7	8	9	10

SUSPECTED TRIGGERS

-
-
-
-

-
-
-
-

SYMPTOMS

RELIEF MEASURES

NOTES

CHRONIC PAIN ASSESSMENT

DATE		DAY	
TIME STARTED		TIME ENDED	
TOTAL DURATION			

RIGHT SIDE   BACK   FRONT   LEFT SIDE

LEFT   RIGHT   RIGHT   LEFT

← Mark the location of the pain

LENGTH OF TIME EXPERIENCING THE PAIN?

< 6 Months			6-12 Months	
1-3 Years			3 Years +	

TYPE OF PAIN

Indescribable		Stabbing		Sharp	
Burning		Aching		Prickly	
Numb		Tingling/ Pins & Needles			
Other					

EXTERNAL ENVIROMENTAL FACTORS

Sun/ Heat		Cold		Windy	
Rain		Aching		Cloudy	
Other					

PAIN SCALE

NO PAIN ⟶ SEVERE PAIN

0	1	2	3	4	5	6	7	8	9	10

SUSPECTED TRIGGERS

-
-
-
-

-
-
-
-

SYMPTOMS

RELIEF MEASURES

NOTES

CHRONIC PAIN ASSESSMENT

DATE		DAY	
TIME STARTED		**TIME ENDED**	
TOTAL DURATION			

RIGHT SIDE   BACK   FRONT   LEFT SIDE

LEFT   RIGHT   RIGHT   LEFT

← Mark the location of the pain

LENGTH OF TIME EXPERIENCING THE PAIN?

< 6 Months		6-12 Months	
1-3 Years		3 Years +	

TYPE OF PAIN

Indescribable		Stabbing		Sharp	
Burning		Aching		Prickly	
Numb		Tingling/ Pins & Needles			
Other					

EXTERNAL ENVIROMENTAL FACTORS

Sun/ Heat		Cold		Windy	
Rain		Aching		Cloudy	
Other					

PAIN SCALE

NO PAIN ————————————————→ SEVERE PAIN

0	1	2	3	4	5	6	7	8	9	10

SUSPECTED TRIGGERS

-
-
-
-

-
-
-
-

SYMPTOMS

RELIEF MEASURES

NOTES

CHRONIC PAIN ASSESSMENT

DATE		DAY	
TIME STARTED		TIME ENDED	
TOTAL DURATION			

RIGHT SIDE   BACK   FRONT   LEFT SIDE

LEFT   RIGHT   RIGHT   LEFT

← ———————   Mark the location of the pain

LENGTH OF TIME EXPERIENCING THE PAIN?

< 6 Months			6-12 Months
1-3 Years			3 Years +

TYPE OF PAIN

Indescribable		Stabbing		Sharp
Burning		Aching		Prickly
Numb		Tingling/ Pins & Needles		
Other				

EXTERNAL ENVIROMENTAL FACTORS

Sun/ Heat		Cold		Windy
Rain		Aching		Cloudy
Other				

PAIN SCALE

NO PAIN ————————————————————→ SEVERE PAIN

0	1	2	3	4	5	6	7	8	9	10

SUSPECTED TRIGGERS

-
-
-
-

-
-
-
-

SYMPTOMS

RELIEF MEASURES

NOTES

CHRONIC PAIN ASSESSMENT

DATE		DAY	
TIME STARTED		**TIME ENDED**	
TOTAL DURATION			

RIGHT SIDE   BACK   FRONT   LEFT SIDE

LEFT RIGHT   RIGHT LEFT

← Mark the location of the pain

LENGTH OF TIME EXPERIENCING THE PAIN?

< 6 Months		6-12 Months	
1-3 Years		3 Years +	

TYPE OF PAIN

Indescribable		Stabbing		Sharp	
Burning		Aching		Prickly	
Numb		Tingling/ Pins & Needles			
Other					

EXTERNAL ENVIROMENTAL FACTORS

Sun/ Heat		Cold		Windy	
Rain		Aching		Cloudy	
Other					

PAIN SCALE

NO PAIN ──────────────────────→ SEVERE PAIN

0	1	2	3	4	5	6	7	8	9	10

SUSPECTED TRIGGERS

-
-
-
-

-
-
-
-

SYMPTOMS

RELIEF MEASURES

NOTES

CHRONIC PAIN ASSESSMENT

DATE		DAY	
TIME STARTED		TIME ENDED	
TOTAL DURATION			

RIGHT SIDE   BACK   FRONT   LEFT SIDE

LEFT RIGHT   RIGHT LEFT

⟵ Mark the location of the pain

LENGTH OF TIME EXPERIENCING THE PAIN?

< 6 Months		6-12 Months	
1-3 Years		3 Years +	

TYPE OF PAIN

Indescribable		Stabbing		Sharp	
Burning		Aching		Prickly	
Numb		Tingling/ Pins & Needles			
Other					

EXTERNAL ENVIROMENTAL FACTORS

Sun/ Heat		Cold		Windy	
Rain		Aching		Cloudy	
Other					

PAIN SCALE

NO PAIN ⟶ SEVERE PAIN

0	1	2	3	4	5	6	7	8	9	10

SUSPECTED TRIGGERS

-
-
-
-

-
-
-
-

SYMPTOMS

RELIEF MEASURES

NOTES

CHRONIC PAIN ASSESSMENT

DATE		DAY	
TIME STARTED		**TIME ENDED**	
TOTAL DURATION			

RIGHT SIDE   BACK   FRONT   LEFT SIDE

LEFT   RIGHT   RIGHT   LEFT

⬅ Mark the location of the pain

LENGTH OF TIME EXPERIENCING THE PAIN?

< 6 Months		6-12 Months	
1-3 Years		3 Years +	

TYPE OF PAIN

Indescribable		Stabbing		Sharp	
Burning		Aching		Prickly	
Numb		Tingling/ Pins & Needles			
Other					

EXTERNAL ENVIROMENTAL FACTORS

Sun/ Heat		Cold		Windy	
Rain		Aching		Cloudy	
Other					

PAIN SCALE

NO PAIN ⟶ SEVERE PAIN

0	1	2	3	4	5	6	7	8	9	10

SUSPECTED TRIGGERS

-
-
-
-

-
-
-
-

SYMPTOMS

RELIEF MEASURES

NOTES

CHRONIC PAIN ASSESSMENT

DATE		DAY	
TIME STARTED		TIME ENDED	
TOTAL DURATION			

RIGHT SIDE   BACK   FRONT   LEFT SIDE

LEFT   RIGHT   RIGHT   LEFT

← Mark the location of the pain

LENGTH OF TIME EXPERIENCING THE PAIN?

< 6 Months			6-12 Months	
1-3 Years			3 Years +	

TYPE OF PAIN

Indescribable		Stabbing		Sharp	
Burning		Aching		Prickly	
Numb		Tingling/ Pins & Needles			
Other					

EXTERNAL ENVIROMENTAL FACTORS

Sun/ Heat		Cold		Windy	
Rain		Aching		Cloudy	
Other					

PAIN SCALE

NO PAIN ⟶ SEVERE PAIN

0	1	2	3	4	5	6	7	8	9	10

SUSPECTED TRIGGERS

-
-
-
-

-
-
-
-

SYMPTOMS

RELIEF MEASURES

NOTES

CHRONIC PAIN ASSESSMENT

DATE		DAY	
TIME STARTED		TIME ENDED	
TOTAL DURATION			

RIGHT SIDE · BACK · FRONT · LEFT SIDE

← Mark the location of the pain

LENGTH OF TIME EXPERIENCING THE PAIN?

< 6 Months		6-12 Months	
1-3 Years		3 Years +	

TYPE OF PAIN

Indescribable		Stabbing		Sharp	
Burning		Aching		Prickly	
Numb		Tingling/ Pins & Needles			
Other					

EXTERNAL ENVIROMENTAL FACTORS

Sun/ Heat		Cold		Windy	
Rain		Aching		Cloudy	
Other					

PAIN SCALE

NO PAIN ———————————————→ SEVERE PAIN

0	1	2	3	4	5	6	7	8	9	10

SUSPECTED TRIGGERS

-
-
-
-

-
-
-
-

SYMPTOMS

RELIEF MEASURES

NOTES

CHRONIC PAIN ASSESSMENT

DATE		DAY	
TIME STARTED		TIME ENDED	
TOTAL DURATION			

RIGHT SIDE   BACK   FRONT   LEFT SIDE

LEFT   RIGHT   RIGHT   LEFT

← ⟵ Mark the location of the pain

LENGTH OF TIME EXPERIENCING THE PAIN?

< 6 Months		6-12 Months	
1-3 Years		3 Years +	

TYPE OF PAIN

Indescribable		Stabbing		Sharp	
Burning		Aching		Prickly	
Numb		Tingling/ Pins & Needles			
Other					

EXTERNAL ENVIROMENTAL FACTORS

Sun/ Heat		Cold		Windy	
Rain		Aching		Cloudy	
Other					

PAIN SCALE

NO PAIN ⟶ SEVERE PAIN

0	1	2	3	4	5	6	7	8	9	10

SUSPECTED TRIGGERS

-
-
-
-
-
-
-
-

SYMPTOMS

RELIEF MEASURES

NOTES

CHRONIC PAIN ASSESSMENT

DATE		DAY	
TIME STARTED		TIME ENDED	
TOTAL DURATION			

RIGHT SIDE   BACK   FRONT   LEFT SIDE

LEFT   RIGHT   RIGHT   LEFT

←   Mark the location of the pain

LENGTH OF TIME EXPERIENCING THE PAIN?

< 6 Months		6-12 Months	
1-3 Years		3 Years +	

TYPE OF PAIN

Indescribable		Stabbing		Sharp	
Burning		Aching		Prickly	
Numb		Tingling/ Pins & Needles			
Other					

EXTERNAL ENVIROMENTAL FACTORS

Sun/ Heat		Cold		Windy	
Rain		Aching		Cloudy	
Other					

PAIN SCALE

NO PAIN   ————————————————→   SEVERE PAIN

0	1	2	3	4	5	6	7	8	9	10

SUSPECTED TRIGGERS

-
-
-
-

-
-
-
-

SYMPTOMS

RELIEF MEASURES

NOTES

CHRONIC PAIN ASSESSMENT

DATE		DAY	
TIME STARTED		TIME ENDED	
TOTAL DURATION			

RIGHT SIDE   BACK   FRONT   LEFT SIDE

LEFT | RIGHT   RIGHT | LEFT

← Mark the location of the pain

LENGTH OF TIME EXPERIENCING THE PAIN?

< 6 Months		6-12 Months	
1-3 Years		3 Years +	

TYPE OF PAIN

Indescribable		Stabbing		Sharp	
Burning		Aching		Prickly	
Numb		Tingling/ Pins & Needles			
Other					

EXTERNAL ENVIROMENTAL FACTORS

Sun/ Heat		Cold		Windy	
Rain		Aching		Cloudy	
Other					

PAIN SCALE

NO PAIN ——————————————————→ SEVERE PAIN

0	1	2	3	4	5	6	7	8	9	10

SUSPECTED TRIGGERS

-
-
-
-

-
-
-
-

SYMPTOMS

RELIEF MEASURES

NOTES

CHRONIC PAIN ASSESSMENT

DATE		DAY	
TIME STARTED		**TIME ENDED**	
TOTAL DURATION			

← Mark the location of the pain

LENGTH OF TIME EXPERIENCING THE PAIN?

< 6 Months		6-12 Months	
1-3 Years		3 Years +	

TYPE OF PAIN

Indescribable		Stabbing		Sharp	
Burning		Aching		Prickly	
Numb		Tingling/ Pins & Needles			
Other					

EXTERNAL ENVIROMENTAL FACTORS

Sun/ Heat		Cold		Windy	
Rain		Aching		Cloudy	
Other					

PAIN SCALE

NO PAIN ——————————————————→ SEVERE PAIN

0	1	2	3	4	5	6	7	8	9	10

SUSPECTED TRIGGERS

-
-
-
-

-
-
-
-

SYMPTOMS

RELIEF MEASURES

NOTES

CHRONIC PAIN ASSESSMENT

DATE		DAY	
TIME STARTED		TIME ENDED	
TOTAL DURATION			

RIGHT SIDE BACK FRONT LEFT SIDE

LEFT RIGHT RIGHT LEFT

← Mark the location of the pain

LENGTH OF TIME EXPERIENCING THE PAIN?

< 6 Months		6-12 Months	
1-3 Years		3 Years +	

TYPE OF PAIN

Indescribable		Stabbing		Sharp	
Burning		Aching		Prickly	
Numb		Tingling/ Pins & Needles			
Other					

EXTERNAL ENVIROMENTAL FACTORS

Sun/ Heat		Cold		Windy	
Rain		Aching		Cloudy	
Other					

PAIN SCALE

NO PAIN ——————————————→ SEVERE PAIN

0	1	2	3	4	5	6	7	8	9	10

SUSPECTED TRIGGERS

-
-
-
-

-
-
-
-

SYMPTOMS

RELIEF MEASURES

NOTES

CHRONIC PAIN ASSESSMENT

DATE		DAY	
TIME STARTED		**TIME ENDED**	
TOTAL DURATION			

RIGHT SIDE   BACK   FRONT   LEFT SIDE

LEFT RIGHT   RIGHT LEFT

←   Mark the location of the pain

LENGTH OF TIME EXPERIENCING THE PAIN?

< 6 Months		6-12 Months	
1-3 Years		3 Years +	

TYPE OF PAIN

Indescribable		Stabbing		Sharp	
Burning		Aching		Prickly	
Numb		Tingling/ Pins & Needles			
Other					

EXTERNAL ENVIROMENTAL FACTORS

Sun/ Heat		Cold		Windy	
Rain		Aching		Cloudy	
Other					

PAIN SCALE

NO PAIN ———————————————————→ SEVERE PAIN

0	1	2	3	4	5	6	7	8	9	10

SUSPECTED TRIGGERS

-
-
-
-

-
-
-
-

SYMPTOMS

RELIEF MEASURES

NOTES

CHRONIC PAIN ASSESSMENT

DATE		DAY	
TIME STARTED		TIME ENDED	
TOTAL DURATION			

← Mark the location of the pain

LENGTH OF TIME EXPERIENCING THE PAIN?

< 6 Months		6-12 Months	
1-3 Years		3 Years +	

TYPE OF PAIN

Indescribable		Stabbing		Sharp	
Burning		Aching		Prickly	
Numb		Tingling/ Pins & Needles			
Other					

EXTERNAL ENVIROMENTAL FACTORS

Sun/ Heat		Cold		Windy	
Rain		Aching		Cloudy	
Other					

PAIN SCALE

NO PAIN ⟶ SEVERE PAIN

0	1	2	3	4	5	6	7	8	9	10

SUSPECTED TRIGGERS

-
-
-
-

-
-
-
-

SYMPTOMS

RELIEF MEASURES

NOTES

CHRONIC PAIN ASSESSMENT

DATE		DAY	
TIME STARTED		TIME ENDED	
TOTAL DURATION			

RIGHT SIDE   BACK   FRONT   LEFT SIDE

Mark the location of the pain ←

LENGTH OF TIME EXPERIENCING THE PAIN?

< 6 Months		6-12 Months	
1-3 Years		3 Years +	

TYPE OF PAIN

Indescribable		Stabbing		Sharp	
Burning		Aching		Prickly	
Numb		Tingling/ Pins & Needles			
Other					

EXTERNAL ENVIROMENTAL FACTORS

Sun/ Heat		Cold		Windy	
Rain		Aching		Cloudy	
Other					

PAIN SCALE

NO PAIN ⟶ SEVERE PAIN

0	1	2	3	4	5	6	7	8	9	10

SUSPECTED TRIGGERS

-
-
-
-

-
-
-
-

SYMPTOMS

RELIEF MEASURES

NOTES

CHRONIC PAIN ASSESSMENT

DATE		DAY	
TIME STARTED		TIME ENDED	
TOTAL DURATION			

RIGHT SIDE   BACK   FRONT   LEFT SIDE

LEFT   RIGHT   RIGHT   LEFT

← Mark the location of the pain

LENGTH OF TIME EXPERIENCING THE PAIN?

< 6 Months		6-12 Months	
1-3 Years		3 Years +	

TYPE OF PAIN

Indescribable		Stabbing		Sharp	
Burning		Aching		Prickly	
Numb		Tingling/ Pins & Needles			
Other					

EXTERNAL ENVIROMENTAL FACTORS

Sun/ Heat		Cold		Windy	
Rain		Aching		Cloudy	
Other					

PAIN SCALE

NO PAIN ———————————————→ SEVERE PAIN

0	1	2	3	4	5	6	7	8	9	10

SUSPECTED TRIGGERS

-
-
-
-

-
-
-
-

SYMPTOMS

RELIEF MEASURES

NOTES

CHRONIC PAIN ASSESSMENT

DATE		DAY	
TIME STARTED		**TIME ENDED**	
TOTAL DURATION			

RIGHT SIDE   BACK   FRONT   LEFT SIDE

LEFT   RIGHT   RIGHT   LEFT

← Mark the location of the pain

LENGTH OF TIME EXPERIENCING THE PAIN?

< 6 Months		6-12 Months	
1-3 Years		3 Years +	

TYPE OF PAIN

Indescribable		Stabbing		Sharp	
Burning		Aching		Prickly	
Numb		Tingling/ Pins & Needles			
Other					

EXTERNAL ENVIROMENTAL FACTORS

Sun/ Heat		Cold		Windy	
Rain		Aching		Cloudy	
Other					

PAIN SCALE

NO PAIN ⟶ SEVERE PAIN

0	1	2	3	4	5	6	7	8	9	10

SUSPECTED TRIGGERS

-
-
-
-

-
-
-
-

SYMPTOMS

RELIEF MEASURES

NOTES

CHRONIC PAIN ASSESSMENT

DATE		DAY	
TIME STARTED		TIME ENDED	
TOTAL DURATION			

RIGHT SIDE BACK FRONT LEFT SIDE

LEFT RIGHT RIGHT LEFT

← _____ Mark the location of the pain

LENGTH OF TIME EXPERIENCING THE PAIN?

< 6 Months		6-12 Months	
1-3 Years		3 Years +	

TYPE OF PAIN

Indescribable		Stabbing		Sharp	
Burning		Aching		Prickly	
Numb		Tingling/ Pins & Needles			
Other					

EXTERNAL ENVIROMENTAL FACTORS

Sun/ Heat		Cold		Windy	
Rain		Aching		Cloudy	
Other					

PAIN SCALE

NO PAIN ——————————————————→ SEVERE PAIN

0	1	2	3	4	5	6	7	8	9	10

SUSPECTED TRIGGERS

-
-
-
-

-
-
-
-

SYMPTOMS

RELIEF MEASURES

NOTES

CHRONIC PAIN ASSESSMENT

DATE		DAY	
TIME STARTED		TIME ENDED	
TOTAL DURATION			

RIGHT SIDE   BACK   FRONT   LEFT SIDE

LEFT RIGHT   RIGHT LEFT

← Mark the location of the pain

LENGTH OF TIME EXPERIENCING THE PAIN?

< 6 Months		6-12 Months
1-3 Years		3 Years +

TYPE OF PAIN

Indescribable		Stabbing		Sharp
Burning		Aching		Prickly
Numb		Tingling/ Pins & Needles		
Other				

EXTERNAL ENVIROMENTAL FACTORS

Sun/ Heat		Cold		Windy
Rain		Aching		Cloudy
Other				

PAIN SCALE

NO PAIN   → SEVERE PAIN

0	1	2	3	4	5	6	7	8	9	10

SUSPECTED TRIGGERS

-
-
-
-

-
-
-
-

SYMPTOMS

RELIEF MEASURES

NOTES

CHRONIC PAIN ASSESSMENT

DATE		DAY	
TIME STARTED		TIME ENDED	
TOTAL DURATION			

RIGHT SIDE   BACK   FRONT   LEFT SIDE

LEFT   RIGHT   RIGHT   LEFT

Mark the location of the pain ←——————

LENGTH OF TIME EXPERIENCING THE PAIN?

< 6 Months		6-12 Months
1-3 Years		3 Years +

TYPE OF PAIN

Indescribable	Stabbing		Sharp	
Burning	Aching		Prickly	
Numb	Tingling/ Pins & Needles			
Other				

EXTERNAL ENVIROMENTAL FACTORS

Sun/ Heat		Cold	Windy
Rain		Aching	Cloudy
Other			

PAIN SCALE

NO PAIN ————————————————————→ SEVERE PAIN

0	1	2	3	4	5	6	7	8	9	10

SUSPECTED TRIGGERS

- _____
- _____
- _____
- _____

- _____
- _____
- _____
- _____

SYMPTOMS

_____
_____
_____
_____
_____
_____
_____
_____

RELIEF MEASURES

_____
_____
_____
_____
_____
_____

NOTES

_____
_____
_____
_____

CHRONIC PAIN ASSESSMENT

DATE		DAY	
TIME STARTED		**TIME ENDED**	
TOTAL DURATION			

RIGHT SIDE   BACK   FRONT   LEFT SIDE

LEFT   RIGHT   RIGHT   LEFT

← Mark the location of the pain

LENGTH OF TIME EXPERIENCING THE PAIN?

< 6 Months		6-12 Months	
1-3 Years		3 Years +	

TYPE OF PAIN

Indescribable		Stabbing		Sharp	
Burning		Aching		Prickly	
Numb		Tingling/ Pins & Needles			
Other					

EXTERNAL ENVIROMENTAL FACTORS

Sun/ Heat		Cold		Windy	
Rain		Aching		Cloudy	
Other					

PAIN SCALE

NO PAIN →→→→→→→→→→→→→→→→→→→→→→→ SEVERE PAIN

0	1	2	3	4	5	6	7	8	9	10

SUSPECTED TRIGGERS

-
-
-
-

-
-
-
-

SYMPTOMS

RELIEF MEASURES

NOTES

CHRONIC PAIN ASSESSMENT

DATE		DAY	
TIME STARTED		TIME ENDED	
TOTAL DURATION			

RIGHT SIDE   BACK   FRONT   LEFT SIDE

LEFT   RIGHT   RIGHT   LEFT

← —————— Mark the location of the pain

LENGTH OF TIME EXPERIENCING THE PAIN?

< 6 Months		6-12 Months	
1-3 Years		3 Years +	

TYPE OF PAIN

Indescribable		Stabbing		Sharp	
Burning		Aching		Prickly	
Numb		Tingling/ Pins & Needles			
Other					

EXTERNAL ENVIROMENTAL FACTORS

Sun/ Heat		Cold		Windy	
Rain		Aching		Cloudy	
Other					

PAIN SCALE

NO PAIN ——————————————————→ SEVERE PAIN

0	1	2	3	4	5	6	7	8	9	10

SUSPECTED TRIGGERS

-
-
-
-

-
-
-
-

SYMPTOMS

RELIEF MEASURES

NOTES

CHRONIC PAIN ASSESSMENT

DATE		DAY	
TIME STARTED		TIME ENDED	
TOTAL DURATION			

← Mark the location of the pain

LENGTH OF TIME EXPERIENCING THE PAIN?

< 6 Months		6-12 Months	
1-3 Years		3 Years +	

TYPE OF PAIN

Indescribable		Stabbing		Sharp	
Burning		Aching		Prickly	
Numb		Tingling/ Pins & Needles			
Other					

EXTERNAL ENVIROMENTAL FACTORS

Sun/ Heat		Cold		Windy	
Rain		Aching		Cloudy	
Other					

PAIN SCALE

NO PAIN ⟶ SEVERE PAIN

0	1	2	3	4	5	6	7	8	9	10

SUSPECTED TRIGGERS

-
-
-
-

-
-
-
-

SYMPTOMS

RELIEF MEASURES

NOTES

CHRONIC PAIN ASSESSMENT

DATE		DAY	
TIME STARTED		TIME ENDED	
TOTAL DURATION			

RIGHT SIDE   BACK   FRONT   LEFT SIDE

← Mark the location of the pain

LENGTH OF TIME EXPERIENCING THE PAIN?

< 6 Months		6-12 Months
1-3 Years		3 Years +

TYPE OF PAIN

Indescribable		Stabbing		Sharp	
Burning		Aching		Prickly	
Numb		Tingling/ Pins & Needles			
Other					

EXTERNAL ENVIROMENTAL FACTORS

Sun/ Heat		Cold		Windy	
Rain		Aching		Cloudy	
Other					

PAIN SCALE

NO PAIN →————————————————————→ SEVERE PAIN

0	1	2	3	4	5	6	7	8	9	10

SUSPECTED TRIGGERS

-       •
-       •
-       •
-       •

SYMPTOMS

RELIEF MEASURES

NOTES

CHRONIC PAIN ASSESSMENT

DATE		DAY	
TIME STARTED		**TIME ENDED**	
TOTAL DURATION			

RIGHT SIDE   BACK   FRONT   LEFT SIDE

LEFT   RIGHT   RIGHT   LEFT

Mark the location of the pain

LENGTH OF TIME EXPERIENCING THE PAIN?

< 6 Months		6-12 Months	
1-3 Years		3 Years +	

TYPE OF PAIN

Indescribable		Stabbing		Sharp	
Burning		Aching		Prickly	
Numb		Tingling/ Pins & Needles			
Other					

EXTERNAL ENVIROMENTAL FACTORS

Sun/ Heat		Cold		Windy	
Rain		Aching		Cloudy	
Other					

PAIN SCALE

NO PAIN ──────────────────────────────────► SEVERE PAIN

0	1	2	3	4	5	6	7	8	9	10

SUSPECTED TRIGGERS

-
-
-
-

-
-
-
-

SYMPTOMS

RELIEF MEASURES

NOTES

CHRONIC PAIN ASSESSMENT

DATE		DAY	
TIME STARTED		TIME ENDED	
TOTAL DURATION			

RIGHT SIDE   BACK   FRONT   LEFT SIDE

LEFT   RIGHT   RIGHT   LEFT

⟵ Mark the location of the pain

LENGTH OF TIME EXPERIENCING THE PAIN?

< 6 Months		6-12 Months
1-3 Years		3 Years +

TYPE OF PAIN

Indescribable	Stabbing	Sharp	
Burning	Aching	Prickly	
Numb	Tingling/ Pins & Needles		
Other			

EXTERNAL ENVIROMENTAL FACTORS

Sun/ Heat	Cold	Windy	
Rain	Aching	Cloudy	
Other			

PAIN SCALE

NO PAIN ⟶ SEVERE PAIN

0	1	2	3	4	5	6	7	8	9	10

SUSPECTED TRIGGERS

-      •
-      •
-      •
-      •

SYMPTOMS

RELIEF MEASURES

NOTES

CHRONIC PAIN ASSESSMENT

DATE		DAY	
TIME STARTED		TIME ENDED	
TOTAL DURATION			

RIGHT SIDE   BACK   FRONT   LEFT SIDE

LEFT   RIGHT   RIGHT   LEFT

← Mark the location of the pain

LENGTH OF TIME EXPERIENCING THE PAIN?

< 6 Months		6-12 Months	
1-3 Years		3 Years +	

TYPE OF PAIN

Indescribable		Stabbing		Sharp	
Burning		Aching		Prickly	
Numb		Tingling/ Pins & Needles			
Other					

EXTERNAL ENVIROMENTAL FACTORS

Sun/ Heat		Cold		Windy	
Rain		Aching		Cloudy	
Other					

PAIN SCALE

NO PAIN ————————————————→ SEVERE PAIN

0	1	2	3	4	5	6	7	8	9	10

SUSPECTED TRIGGERS

-
-
-
-

-
-
-
-

SYMPTOMS

RELIEF MEASURES

NOTES

CHRONIC PAIN ASSESSMENT

DATE		DAY	
TIME STARTED		TIME ENDED	
TOTAL DURATION			

Mark the location of the pain

LENGTH OF TIME EXPERIENCING THE PAIN?

< 6 Months		6-12 Months
1-3 Years		3 Years +

TYPE OF PAIN

Indescribable	Stabbing	Sharp
Burning	Aching	Prickly
Numb	Tingling/ Pins & Needles	
Other		

EXTERNAL ENVIROMENTAL FACTORS

Sun/ Heat	Cold	Windy
Rain	Aching	Cloudy
Other		

PAIN SCALE

NO PAIN ⟶ SEVERE PAIN

0	1	2	3	4	5	6	7	8	9	10

SUSPECTED TRIGGERS

-
-
-
-

-
-
-
-

SYMPTOMS

RELIEF MEASURES

NOTES

CHRONIC PAIN ASSESSMENT

DATE		DAY	
TIME STARTED		TIME ENDED	
TOTAL DURATION			

RIGHT SIDE   BACK   FRONT   LEFT SIDE

LEFT   RIGHT   RIGHT   LEFT

←   Mark the location of the pain

LENGTH OF TIME EXPERIENCING THE PAIN?

< 6 Months		6-12 Months
1-3 Years		3 Years +

TYPE OF PAIN

Indescribable	Stabbing	Sharp
Burning	Aching	Prickly
Numb	Tingling/ Pins & Needles	
Other		

EXTERNAL ENVIROMENTAL FACTORS

Sun/ Heat		Cold	Windy
Rain		Aching	Cloudy
Other			

PAIN SCALE

NO PAIN ⟶ SEVERE PAIN

0	1	2	3	4	5	6	7	8	9	10

SUSPECTED TRIGGERS

-      •
-      •
-      •
-      •

SYMPTOMS

RELIEF MEASURES

NOTES

CHRONIC PAIN ASSESSMENT

DATE		DAY	
TIME STARTED		TIME ENDED	
TOTAL DURATION			

RIGHT SIDE   BACK   FRONT   LEFT SIDE

LEFT   RIGHT   RIGHT   LEFT

← Mark the location of the pain

LENGTH OF TIME EXPERIENCING THE PAIN?

< 6 Months			6-12 Months
1-3 Years			3 Years +

TYPE OF PAIN

Indescribable		Stabbing		Sharp	
Burning		Aching		Prickly	
Numb		Tingling/ Pins & Needles			
Other					

EXTERNAL ENVIROMENTAL FACTORS

Sun/ Heat			Cold	Windy
Rain			Aching	Cloudy
Other				

PAIN SCALE

NO PAIN ——————————————→ SEVERE PAIN

0	1	2	3	4	5	6	7	8	9	10

SUSPECTED TRIGGERS

-
-
-
-

-
-
-
-

SYMPTOMS

RELIEF MEASURES

NOTES

CHRONIC PAIN ASSESSMENT

DATE		DAY	
TIME STARTED		TIME ENDED	
TOTAL DURATION			

RIGHT SIDE   BACK   FRONT   LEFT SIDE

LEFT   RIGHT   RIGHT   LEFT

←   Mark the location of the pain

LENGTH OF TIME EXPERIENCING THE PAIN?

< 6 Months		6-12 Months
1-3 Years		3 Years +

TYPE OF PAIN

Indescribable	Stabbing	Sharp
Burning	Aching	Prickly
Numb	Tingling/ Pins & Needles	
Other		

EXTERNAL ENVIROMENTAL FACTORS

Sun/ Heat	Cold	Windy
Rain	Aching	Cloudy
Other		

PAIN SCALE

NO PAIN ⟶ SEVERE PAIN

0	1	2	3	4	5	6	7	8	9	10

SUSPECTED TRIGGERS

-
-
-
-

-
-
-
-

SYMPTOMS

RELIEF MEASURES

NOTES

CHRONIC PAIN ASSESSMENT

DATE		DAY	
TIME STARTED		TIME ENDED	
TOTAL DURATION			

RIGHT SIDE   BACK   FRONT   LEFT SIDE

LEFT   RIGHT   RIGHT   LEFT

← Mark the location of the pain

LENGTH OF TIME EXPERIENCING THE PAIN?

< 6 Months		6-12 Months
1-3 Years		3 Years +

TYPE OF PAIN

Indescribable		Stabbing		Sharp
Burning		Aching		Prickly
Numb		Tingling/ Pins & Needles		
Other				

EXTERNAL ENVIROMENTAL FACTORS

Sun/ Heat		Cold		Windy
Rain		Aching		Cloudy
Other				

PAIN SCALE

NO PAIN ————————————————→ SEVERE PAIN

0	1	2	3	4	5	6	7	8	9	10

SUSPECTED TRIGGERS

-
-
-
-

-
-
-
-

SYMPTOMS

RELIEF MEASURES

NOTES

CHRONIC PAIN ASSESSMENT

DATE		DAY	
TIME STARTED		TIME ENDED	
TOTAL DURATION			

RIGHT SIDE   BACK   FRONT   LEFT SIDE

← ─────── Mark the location of the pain

LENGTH OF TIME EXPERIENCING THE PAIN?

< 6 Months		6-12 Months
1-3 Years		3 Years +

TYPE OF PAIN

Indescribable	Stabbing	Sharp	
Burning	Aching	Prickly	
Numb	Tingling/ Pins & Needles		
Other			

EXTERNAL ENVIROMENTAL FACTORS

Sun/ Heat		Cold	Windy
Rain		Aching	Cloudy
Other			

PAIN SCALE

NO PAIN ──────────────────────→ SEVERE PAIN

0	1	2	3	4	5	6	7	8	9	10

SUSPECTED TRIGGERS

-
-
-
-

-
-
-
-

SYMPTOMS

RELIEF MEASURES

NOTES

CHRONIC PAIN ASSESSMENT

DATE		DAY	
TIME STARTED		TIME ENDED	
TOTAL DURATION			

RIGHT SIDE   BACK   FRONT   LEFT SIDE

LEFT   RIGHT   RIGHT   LEFT

Mark the location of the pain

LENGTH OF TIME EXPERIENCING THE PAIN?

< 6 Months		6-12 Months	
1-3 Years		3 Years +	

TYPE OF PAIN

Indescribable		Stabbing		Sharp	
Burning		Aching		Prickly	
Numb		Tingling/ Pins & Needles			
Other					

EXTERNAL ENVIROMENTAL FACTORS

Sun/ Heat		Cold		Windy	
Rain		Aching		Cloudy	
Other					

PAIN SCALE

NO PAIN ⟶ SEVERE PAIN

0	1	2	3	4	5	6	7	8	9	10

SUSPECTED TRIGGERS

- _____   • _____
- _____   • _____
- _____   • _____
- _____   • _____

SYMPTOMS

_____
_____
_____
_____
_____
_____
_____
_____

RELIEF MEASURES

_____
_____
_____
_____
_____
_____

NOTES

_____
_____
_____
_____
_____

CHRONIC PAIN ASSESSMENT

DATE		DAY	
TIME STARTED		TIME ENDED	
TOTAL DURATION			

RIGHT SIDE — BACK — FRONT — LEFT SIDE

← Mark the location of the pain

LENGTH OF TIME EXPERIENCING THE PAIN?

< 6 Months		6-12 Months
1-3 Years		3 Years +

TYPE OF PAIN

Indescribable	Stabbing	Sharp
Burning	Aching	Prickly
Numb	Tingling/ Pins & Needles	
Other		

EXTERNAL ENVIROMENTAL FACTORS

Sun/ Heat		Cold	Windy
Rain		Aching	Cloudy
Other			

PAIN SCALE

NO PAIN ⟶ SEVERE PAIN

0	1	2	3	4	5	6	7	8	9	10

SUSPECTED TRIGGERS

-
-
-
-

-
-
-
-

SYMPTOMS

RELIEF MEASURES

NOTES

CHRONIC PAIN ASSESSMENT

DATE		DAY	
TIME STARTED		TIME ENDED	
TOTAL DURATION			

RIGHT SIDE　　BACK　　　FRONT　　LEFT SIDE

LEFT　RIGHT　RIGHT　LEFT

← Mark the location of the pain

LENGTH OF TIME EXPERIENCING THE PAIN?

< 6 Months		6-12 Months
1-3 Years		3 Years +

TYPE OF PAIN

Indescribable	Stabbing	Sharp
Burning	Aching	Prickly
Numb	Tingling/ Pins & Needles	
Other		

EXTERNAL ENVIROMENTAL FACTORS

Sun/ Heat	Cold	Windy
Rain	Aching	Cloudy
Other		

PAIN SCALE

NO PAIN ——————————————→ SEVERE PAIN

0	1	2	3	4	5	6	7	8	9	10

SUSPECTED TRIGGERS

-
-
-
-

-
-
-
-

SYMPTOMS

RELIEF MEASURES

NOTES

CHRONIC PAIN ASSESSMENT

DATE		DAY	
TIME STARTED		**TIME ENDED**	
TOTAL DURATION			

RIGHT SIDE   BACK   FRONT   LEFT SIDE

LEFT   RIGHT   RIGHT   LEFT

← Mark the location of the pain

LENGTH OF TIME EXPERIENCING THE PAIN?

< 6 Months		6-12 Months
1-3 Years		3 Years +

TYPE OF PAIN

Indescribable		Stabbing		Sharp	
Burning		Aching		Prickly	
Numb		Tingling/ Pins & Needles			
Other					

EXTERNAL ENVIROMENTAL FACTORS

Sun/ Heat		Cold		Windy	
Rain		Aching		Cloudy	
Other					

PAIN SCALE

NO PAIN ————————————————→ SEVERE PAIN

0	1	2	3	4	5	6	7	8	9	10

SUSPECTED TRIGGERS

-
-
-
-

-
-
-
-

SYMPTOMS

RELIEF MEASURES

NOTES

CHRONIC PAIN ASSESSMENT

DATE		DAY	
TIME STARTED		**TIME ENDED**	
TOTAL DURATION			

RIGHT SIDE   BACK   FRONT   LEFT SIDE

LEFT RIGHT   RIGHT LEFT

← Mark the location of the pain

LENGTH OF TIME EXPERIENCING THE PAIN?

< 6 Months		6-12 Months
1-3 Years		3 Years +

TYPE OF PAIN

Indescribable	Stabbing	Sharp
Burning	Aching	Prickly
Numb	Tingling/ Pins & Needles	
Other		

EXTERNAL ENVIROMENTAL FACTORS

Sun/ Heat	Cold	Windy
Rain	Aching	Cloudy
Other		

PAIN SCALE

NO PAIN ————————————————→ SEVERE PAIN

0	1	2	3	4	5	6	7	8	9	10

SUSPECTED TRIGGERS

-
-
-
-

-
-
-
-

SYMPTOMS

RELIEF MEASURES

NOTES

CHRONIC PAIN ASSESSMENT

DATE		DAY	
TIME STARTED		TIME ENDED	
TOTAL DURATION			

RIGHT SIDE   BACK   FRONT   LEFT SIDE

← Mark the location of the pain

LENGTH OF TIME EXPERIENCING THE PAIN?

< 6 Months		6-12 Months	
1-3 Years		3 Years +	

TYPE OF PAIN

Indescribable		Stabbing		Sharp	
Burning		Aching		Prickly	
Numb		Tingling/ Pins & Needles			
Other					

EXTERNAL ENVIROMENTAL FACTORS

Sun/ Heat		Cold		Windy	
Rain		Aching		Cloudy	
Other					

PAIN SCALE

NO PAIN ⟶ SEVERE PAIN

0	1	2	3	4	5	6	7	8	9	10

SUSPECTED TRIGGERS

•	•
•	•
•	•
•	•

SYMPTOMS

RELIEF MEASURES

NOTES

CHRONIC PAIN ASSESSMENT

DATE		DAY	
TIME STARTED		TIME ENDED	
TOTAL DURATION			

RIGHT SIDE | BACK | FRONT | LEFT SIDE

← ——————— Mark the location of the pain

LENGTH OF TIME EXPERIENCING THE PAIN?

< 6 Months		6-12 Months
1-3 Years		3 Years +

TYPE OF PAIN

Indescribable		Stabbing		Sharp
Burning		Aching		Prickly
Numb		Tingling/ Pins & Needles		
Other				

EXTERNAL ENVIROMENTAL FACTORS

Sun/ Heat		Cold		Windy
Rain		Aching		Cloudy
Other				

PAIN SCALE

NO PAIN ————————————————→ SEVERE PAIN

0	1	2	3	4	5	6	7	8	9	10

SUSPECTED TRIGGERS

-
-
-
-

-
-
-
-

SYMPTOMS

RELIEF MEASURES

NOTES

CHRONIC PAIN ASSESSMENT

DATE		DAY	
TIME STARTED		TIME ENDED	
TOTAL DURATION			

RIGHT SIDE   BACK   FRONT   LEFT SIDE

← Mark the location of the pain

LENGTH OF TIME EXPERIENCING THE PAIN?

< 6 Months		6-12 Months	
1-3 Years		3 Years +	

TYPE OF PAIN

Indescribable		Stabbing		Sharp	
Burning		Aching		Prickly	
Numb		Tingling/ Pins & Needles			
Other					

EXTERNAL ENVIROMENTAL FACTORS

Sun/ Heat		Cold		Windy	
Rain		Aching		Cloudy	
Other					

PAIN SCALE

NO PAIN ——————————————→ SEVERE PAIN

0	1	2	3	4	5	6	7	8	9	10

SUSPECTED TRIGGERS

•	•
•	•
•	•
•	•

SYMPTOMS

RELIEF MEASURES

NOTES

CHRONIC PAIN ASSESSMENT

DATE		DAY	
TIME STARTED		TIME ENDED	
TOTAL DURATION			

RIGHT SIDE   BACK   FRONT   LEFT SIDE

LEFT RIGHT   RIGHT LEFT

← ——— Mark the location of the pain

LENGTH OF TIME EXPERIENCING THE PAIN?

< 6 Months		6-12 Months
1-3 Years		3 Years +

TYPE OF PAIN

Indescribable		Stabbing		Sharp
Burning		Aching		Prickly
Numb		Tingling/ Pins & Needles		
Other				

EXTERNAL ENVIROMENTAL FACTORS

Sun/ Heat		Cold		Windy
Rain		Aching		Cloudy
Other				

PAIN SCALE

NO PAIN ——————————————————→ SEVERE PAIN

0	1	2	3	4	5	6	7	8	9	10

SUSPECTED TRIGGERS

-         •
-         •
-         •
-         •

SYMPTOMS

RELIEF MEASURES

NOTES

CHRONIC PAIN ASSESSMENT

DATE		DAY	
TIME STARTED		**TIME ENDED**	
TOTAL DURATION			

RIGHT SIDE   BACK   FRONT   LEFT SIDE

LEFT   RIGHT   RIGHT   LEFT

← Mark the location of the pain

LENGTH OF TIME EXPERIENCING THE PAIN?

< 6 Months		6-12 Months
1-3 Years		3 Years +

TYPE OF PAIN

Indescribable	Stabbing	Sharp
Burning	Aching	Prickly
Numb	Tingling/ Pins & Needles	
Other		

EXTERNAL ENVIROMENTAL FACTORS

Sun/ Heat	Cold	Windy
Rain	Aching	Cloudy
Other		

PAIN SCALE
NO PAIN ⟶ SEVERE PAIN

0	1	2	3	4	5	6	7	8	9	10

SUSPECTED TRIGGERS

-
-
-
-

SYMPTOMS

RELIEF MEASURES

NOTES

CHRONIC PAIN ASSESSMENT

DATE		DAY	
TIME STARTED		TIME ENDED	
TOTAL DURATION			

RIGHT SIDE BACK FRONT LEFT SIDE

LEFT RIGHT RIGHT LEFT

← Mark the location of the pain

LENGTH OF TIME EXPERIENCING THE PAIN?

< 6 Months		6-12 Months
1-3 Years		3 Years +

TYPE OF PAIN

Indescribable	Stabbing	Sharp
Burning	Aching	Prickly
Numb	Tingling/ Pins & Needles	
Other		

EXTERNAL ENVIROMENTAL FACTORS

Sun/ Heat	Cold	Windy
Rain	Aching	Cloudy
Other		

PAIN SCALE

NO PAIN ———————————————→ SEVERE PAIN

0	1	2	3	4	5	6	7	8	9	10

SUSPECTED TRIGGERS

-
-
-
-

-
-
-
-

SYMPTOMS

RELIEF MEASURES

NOTES

CHRONIC PAIN ASSESSMENT

DATE		DAY	
TIME STARTED		**TIME ENDED**	
TOTAL DURATION			

RIGHT SIDE   BACK   FRONT   LEFT SIDE

LEFT RIGHT   RIGHT LEFT

← Mark the location of the pain

LENGTH OF TIME EXPERIENCING THE PAIN?

< 6 Months		6-12 Months
1-3 Years		3 Years +

TYPE OF PAIN

Indescribable	Stabbing		Sharp	
Burning	Aching		Prickly	
Numb	Tingling/ Pins & Needles			
Other				

EXTERNAL ENVIROMENTAL FACTORS

Sun/ Heat		Cold		Windy
Rain		Aching		Cloudy
Other				

PAIN SCALE

NO PAIN ⟶ SEVERE PAIN

0	1	2	3	4	5	6	7	8	9	10

SUSPECTED TRIGGERS

-
-
-
-

-
-
-
-

SYMPTOMS

RELIEF MEASURES

NOTES

CHRONIC PAIN ASSESSMENT

DATE		DAY	
TIME STARTED		TIME ENDED	
TOTAL DURATION			

RIGHT SIDE   BACK   FRONT   LEFT SIDE

LEFT   RIGHT   RIGHT   LEFT

← Mark the location of the pain

LENGTH OF TIME EXPERIENCING THE PAIN?

< 6 Months		6-12 Months
1-3 Years		3 Years +

TYPE OF PAIN

Indescribable	Stabbing	Sharp
Burning	Aching	Prickly
Numb	Tingling/ Pins & Needles	
Other		

EXTERNAL ENVIROMENTAL FACTORS

Sun/ Heat		Cold	Windy
Rain		Aching	Cloudy
Other			

PAIN SCALE

NO PAIN ──────────────────────────→ SEVERE PAIN

0	1	2	3	4	5	6	7	8	9	10

SUSPECTED TRIGGERS

-
-
-
-

-
-
-
-

SYMPTOMS

RELIEF MEASURES

NOTES

CHRONIC PAIN ASSESSMENT

DATE		DAY		
TIME STARTED		**TIME ENDED**		
TOTAL DURATION				

RIGHT SIDE   BACK   FRONT   LEFT SIDE

LEFT   RIGHT   RIGHT   LEFT

← Mark the location of the pain

LENGTH OF TIME EXPERIENCING THE PAIN?

< 6 Months		6-12 Months
1-3 Years		3 Years +

TYPE OF PAIN

Indescribable	Stabbing		Sharp
Burning	Aching		Prickly
Numb	Tingling/ Pins & Needles		
Other			

EXTERNAL ENVIROMENTAL FACTORS

Sun/ Heat		Cold		Windy
Rain		Aching		Cloudy
Other				

PAIN SCALE

NO PAIN ——————————————————→ SEVERE PAIN

0	1	2	3	4	5	6	7	8	9	10

SUSPECTED TRIGGERS

-
-
-
-

-
-
-
-

SYMPTOMS

RELIEF MEASURES

NOTES

CHRONIC PAIN ASSESSMENT

DATE		DAY	
TIME STARTED		TIME ENDED	
TOTAL DURATION			

RIGHT SIDE   BACK   FRONT   LEFT SIDE

Mark the location of the pain

LENGTH OF TIME EXPERIENCING THE PAIN?

< 6 Months		6-12 Months
1-3 Years		3 Years +

TYPE OF PAIN

Indescribable	Stabbing	Sharp
Burning	Aching	Prickly
Numb	Tingling/ Pins & Needles	
Other		

EXTERNAL ENVIROMENTAL FACTORS

Sun/ Heat	Cold	Windy
Rain	Aching	Cloudy
Other		

PAIN SCALE

NO PAIN ————————————————————→ SEVERE PAIN

0	1	2	3	4	5	6	7	8	9	10

SUSPECTED TRIGGERS

-
-
-
-

-
-
-
-

SYMPTOMS

RELIEF MEASURES

NOTES

CHRONIC PAIN ASSESSMENT

DATE		DAY	
TIME STARTED		TIME ENDED	
TOTAL DURATION			

RIGHT SIDE   BACK   FRONT   LEFT SIDE

LEFT RIGHT RIGHT LEFT

←   Mark the location of the pain

LENGTH OF TIME EXPERIENCING THE PAIN?

< 6 Months			6-12 Months
1-3 Years			3 Years +

TYPE OF PAIN

Indescribable	Stabbing	Sharp
Burning	Aching	Prickly
Numb	Tingling/ Pins & Needles	
Other		

EXTERNAL ENVIROMENTAL FACTORS

Sun/ Heat		Cold	Windy
Rain		Aching	Cloudy
Other			

PAIN SCALE

NO PAIN   ⟶   SEVERE PAIN

0	1	2	3	4	5	6	7	8	9	10

SUSPECTED TRIGGERS

-        •
-        •
-        •
-        •

SYMPTOMS

RELIEF MEASURES

NOTES

CHRONIC PAIN ASSESSMENT

DATE		DAY	
TIME STARTED		TIME ENDED	
TOTAL DURATION			

RIGHT SIDE   BACK   FRONT   LEFT SIDE

LEFT   RIGHT   RIGHT   LEFT

← Mark the location of the pain

LENGTH OF TIME EXPERIENCING THE PAIN?

< 6 Months		6-12 Months
1-3 Years		3 Years +

TYPE OF PAIN

Indescribable	Stabbing		Sharp
Burning	Aching		Prickly
Numb	Tingling/ Pins & Needles		
Other			

EXTERNAL ENVIROMENTAL FACTORS

Sun/ Heat		Cold	Windy
Rain		Aching	Cloudy
Other			

PAIN SCALE

NO PAIN ————————————————→ SEVERE PAIN

0	1	2	3	4	5	6	7	8	9	10

SUSPECTED TRIGGERS

-
-
-
-

-
-
-
-

SYMPTOMS

RELIEF MEASURES

NOTES

CHRONIC PAIN ASSESSMENT

DATE		DAY		
TIME STARTED		**TIME ENDED**		
TOTAL DURATION				

RIGHT SIDE BACK FRONT LEFT SIDE

LEFT RIGHT RIGHT LEFT

Mark the location of the pain

LENGTH OF TIME EXPERIENCING THE PAIN?

< 6 Months		6-12 Months
1-3 Years		3 Years +

TYPE OF PAIN

Indescribable	Stabbing	Sharp
Burning	Aching	Prickly
Numb	Tingling/ Pins & Needles	
Other		

EXTERNAL ENVIROMENTAL FACTORS

Sun/ Heat		Cold	Windy
Rain		Aching	Cloudy
Other			

PAIN SCALE

NO PAIN ⟶ SEVERE PAIN

0	1	2	3	4	5	6	7	8	9	10

SUSPECTED TRIGGERS

-
-
-
-

-
-
-
-

SYMPTOMS

RELIEF MEASURES

NOTES

CHRONIC PAIN ASSESSMENT

DATE		DAY	
TIME STARTED		TIME ENDED	
TOTAL DURATION			

RIGHT SIDE   BACK   FRONT   LEFT SIDE

LEFT   RIGHT   RIGHT   LEFT

← ——————— Mark the location of the pain

LENGTH OF TIME EXPERIENCING THE PAIN?

< 6 Months		6-12 Months
1-3 Years		3 Years +

TYPE OF PAIN

Indescribable	Stabbing	Sharp
Burning	Aching	Prickly
Numb	Tingling/ Pins & Needles	
Other		

EXTERNAL ENVIROMENTAL FACTORS

Sun/ Heat	Cold	Windy
Rain	Aching	Cloudy
Other		

PAIN SCALE

NO PAIN ————————————————————→ SEVERE PAIN

0	1	2	3	4	5	6	7	8	9	10

SUSPECTED TRIGGERS

•	•
•	•
•	•
•	•

SYMPTOMS

RELIEF MEASURES

NOTES

CHRONIC PAIN ASSESSMENT

DATE		DAY	
TIME STARTED		TIME ENDED	
TOTAL DURATION			

RIGHT SIDE   BACK   FRONT   LEFT SIDE

LEFT   RIGHT   RIGHT   LEFT

← Mark the location of the pain

LENGTH OF TIME EXPERIENCING THE PAIN?

< 6 Months		6-12 Months	
1-3 Years		3 Years +	

TYPE OF PAIN

Indescribable		Stabbing		Sharp	
Burning		Aching		Prickly	
Numb		Tingling/ Pins & Needles			
Other					

EXTERNAL ENVIROMENTAL FACTORS

Sun/ Heat		Cold		Windy	
Rain		Aching		Cloudy	
Other					

PAIN SCALE

NO PAIN ————————————————→ SEVERE PAIN

0	1	2	3	4	5	6	7	8	9	10

SUSPECTED TRIGGERS

-
-
-
-

SYMPTOMS

RELIEF MEASURES

NOTES

CHRONIC PAIN ASSESSMENT

DATE		DAY	
TIME STARTED		TIME ENDED	
TOTAL DURATION			

RIGHT SIDE   BACK   FRONT   LEFT SIDE

LEFT RIGHT   RIGHT LEFT

←   Mark the location of the pain

LENGTH OF TIME EXPERIENCING THE PAIN?

< 6 Months		6-12 Months
1-3 Years		3 Years +

TYPE OF PAIN

Indescribable	Stabbing		Sharp
Burning	Aching		Prickly
Numb	Tingling/ Pins & Needles		
Other			

EXTERNAL ENVIROMENTAL FACTORS

Sun/ Heat		Cold	Windy
Rain		Aching	Cloudy
Other			

PAIN SCALE

NO PAIN ————————————————————→ SEVERE PAIN

0	1	2	3	4	5	6	7	8	9	10

SUSPECTED TRIGGERS

-
-
-
-

-
-
-
-

SYMPTOMS

RELIEF MEASURES

NOTES

CHRONIC PAIN ASSESSMENT

DATE		DAY	
TIME STARTED		TIME ENDED	
TOTAL DURATION			

RIGHT SIDE   BACK   FRONT   LEFT SIDE

LEFT   RIGHT   RIGHT   LEFT

← Mark the location of the pain

LENGTH OF TIME EXPERIENCING THE PAIN?

< 6 Months		6-12 Months
1-3 Years		3 Years +

TYPE OF PAIN

Indescribable		Stabbing		Sharp	
Burning		Aching		Prickly	
Numb		Tingling/ Pins & Needles			
Other					

EXTERNAL ENVIROMENTAL FACTORS

Sun/ Heat		Cold		Windy	
Rain		Aching		Cloudy	
Other					

PAIN SCALE

NO PAIN ——————————————→ SEVERE PAIN

0	1	2	3	4	5	6	7	8	9	10

SUSPECTED TRIGGERS

-
-
-
-

-
-
-
-

SYMPTOMS

RELIEF MEASURES

NOTES

CHRONIC PAIN ASSESSMENT

DATE		DAY	
TIME STARTED		TIME ENDED	
TOTAL DURATION			

RIGHT SIDE · BACK · FRONT · LEFT SIDE

← Mark the location of the pain

LENGTH OF TIME EXPERIENCING THE PAIN?

< 6 Months		6-12 Months
1-3 Years		3 Years +

TYPE OF PAIN

Indescribable	Stabbing	Sharp
Burning	Aching	Prickly
Numb	Tingling/ Pins & Needles	
Other		

EXTERNAL ENVIROMENTAL FACTORS

Sun/ Heat	Cold	Windy
Rain	Aching	Cloudy
Other		

PAIN SCALE

NO PAIN ————————————————→ SEVERE PAIN

0	1	2	3	4	5	6	7	8	9	10

SUSPECTED TRIGGERS

-
-
-
-

-
-
-
-

SYMPTOMS

RELIEF MEASURES

NOTES

CHRONIC PAIN ASSESSMENT

DATE		**DAY**	
TIME STARTED		**TIME ENDED**	
TOTAL DURATION			

RIGHT SIDE   BACK   FRONT   LEFT SIDE

LEFT RIGHT   RIGHT LEFT

← Mark the location of the pain

LENGTH OF TIME EXPERIENCING THE PAIN?

< 6 Months		6-12 Months	
1-3 Years		3 Years +	

TYPE OF PAIN

Indescribable		Stabbing		Sharp	
Burning		Aching		Prickly	
Numb		Tingling/ Pins & Needles			
Other					

EXTERNAL ENVIROMENTAL FACTORS

Sun/ Heat		Cold		Windy	
Rain		Aching		Cloudy	
Other					

PAIN SCALE

NO PAIN   ————————————————→ SEVERE PAIN

0	1	2	3	4	5	6	7	8	9	10

SUSPECTED TRIGGERS

•	•
•	•
•	•
•	•

SYMPTOMS

RELIEF MEASURES

NOTES

CHRONIC PAIN ASSESSMENT

DATE		DAY	
TIME STARTED		**TIME ENDED**	
TOTAL DURATION			

RIGHT SIDE   BACK   FRONT   LEFT SIDE

LEFT RIGHT   RIGHT LEFT

← ———————— Mark the location of the pain

LENGTH OF TIME EXPERIENCING THE PAIN?

< 6 Months		6-12 Months
1-3 Years		3 Years +

TYPE OF PAIN

Indescribable	Stabbing	Sharp	
Burning	Aching	Prickly	
Numb	Tingling/ Pins & Needles		
Other			

EXTERNAL ENVIROMENTAL FACTORS

Sun/ Heat		Cold	Windy
Rain		Aching	Cloudy
Other			

PAIN SCALE

NO PAIN ————————————————→ SEVERE PAIN

0	1	2	3	4	5	6	7	8	9	10

SUSPECTED TRIGGERS

•	•
•	•
•	•
•	•

SYMPTOMS

RELIEF MEASURES

NOTES

CHRONIC PAIN ASSESSMENT

DATE		DAY	
TIME STARTED		**TIME ENDED**	
TOTAL DURATION			

RIGHT SIDE   BACK   FRONT   LEFT SIDE

LEFT   RIGHT   RIGHT   LEFT

← Mark the location of the pain

LENGTH OF TIME EXPERIENCING THE PAIN?

< 6 Months		6-12 Months	
1-3 Years		3 Years +	

TYPE OF PAIN

Indescribable		Stabbing		Sharp	
Burning		Aching		Prickly	
Numb		Tingling/ Pins & Needles			
Other					

EXTERNAL ENVIROMENTAL FACTORS

Sun/ Heat		Cold		Windy	
Rain		Aching		Cloudy	
Other					

PAIN SCALE

NO PAIN ————————————————→ SEVERE PAIN

0	1	2	3	4	5	6	7	8	9	10

SUSPECTED TRIGGERS

- _____   - _____
- _____   - _____
- _____   - _____
- _____   - _____

SYMPTOMS

_____
_____
_____
_____
_____
_____
_____
_____

RELIEF MEASURES

_____
_____
_____
_____
_____
_____

NOTES

_____
_____
_____
_____
_____

CHRONIC PAIN ASSESSMENT

DATE		DAY	
TIME STARTED		TIME ENDED	
TOTAL DURATION			

RIGHT SIDE   BACK   FRONT   LEFT SIDE

LEFT   RIGHT   RIGHT   LEFT

← ——— Mark the location of the pain

LENGTH OF TIME EXPERIENCING THE PAIN?

< 6 Months		6-12 Months
1-3 Years		3 Years +

TYPE OF PAIN

Indescribable	Stabbing	Sharp
Burning	Aching	Prickly
Numb	Tingling/ Pins & Needles	
Other		

EXTERNAL ENVIROMENTAL FACTORS

Sun/ Heat	Cold	Windy
Rain	Aching	Cloudy
Other		

PAIN SCALE

NO PAIN ——————————————→ SEVERE PAIN

0	1	2	3	4	5	6	7	8	9	10

SUSPECTED TRIGGERS

-
-
-
-

-
-
-
-

SYMPTOMS

RELIEF MEASURES

NOTES

CHRONIC PAIN ASSESSMENT

DATE		DAY	
TIME STARTED		TIME ENDED	
TOTAL DURATION			

RIGHT SIDE BACK FRONT LEFT SIDE

← Mark the location of the pain

LENGTH OF TIME EXPERIENCING THE PAIN?

< 6 Months		6-12 Months	
1-3 Years		3 Years +	

TYPE OF PAIN

Indescribable		Stabbing		Sharp	
Burning		Aching		Prickly	
Numb		Tingling/ Pins & Needles			
Other					

EXTERNAL ENVIROMENTAL FACTORS

Sun/ Heat		Cold		Windy	
Rain		Aching		Cloudy	
Other					

PAIN SCALE

NO PAIN ——————————————→ SEVERE PAIN

0	1	2	3	4	5	6	7	8	9	10

SUSPECTED TRIGGERS

-
-
-
-

-
-
-
-

SYMPTOMS

RELIEF MEASURES

NOTES

CHRONIC PAIN ASSESSMENT

DATE		DAY	
TIME STARTED		TIME ENDED	
TOTAL DURATION			

RIGHT SIDE   BACK   FRONT   LEFT SIDE

LEFT   RIGHT   RIGHT   LEFT

← Mark the location of the pain

LENGTH OF TIME EXPERIENCING THE PAIN?

< 6 Months		6-12 Months	
1-3 Years		3 Years +	

TYPE OF PAIN

Indescribable		Stabbing		Sharp	
Burning		Aching		Prickly	
Numb		Tingling/ Pins & Needles			
Other					

EXTERNAL ENVIROMENTAL FACTORS

Sun/ Heat		Cold		Windy	
Rain		Aching		Cloudy	
Other					

PAIN SCALE

NO PAIN ──────────────────────→ SEVERE PAIN

0	1	2	3	4	5	6	7	8	9	10

SUSPECTED TRIGGERS

-
-
-
-

-
-
-
-

SYMPTOMS

RELIEF MEASURES

NOTES

CHRONIC PAIN ASSESSMENT

DATE		DAY	
TIME STARTED		**TIME ENDED**	
TOTAL DURATION			

RIGHT SIDE   BACK   FRONT   LEFT SIDE

LEFT   RIGHT   RIGHT   LEFT

←   Mark the location of the pain

LENGTH OF TIME EXPERIENCING THE PAIN?

< 6 Months		6-12 Months
1-3 Years		3 Years +

TYPE OF PAIN

Indescribable		Stabbing		Sharp
Burning		Aching		Prickly
Numb		Tingling/ Pins & Needles		
Other				

EXTERNAL ENVIROMENTAL FACTORS

Sun/ Heat		Cold		Windy
Rain		Aching		Cloudy
Other				

PAIN SCALE

NO PAIN   ⟶   SEVERE PAIN

0	1	2	3	4	5	6	7	8	9	10

SUSPECTED TRIGGERS

-
-
-
-

-
-
-
-

SYMPTOMS

RELIEF MEASURES

NOTES

CHRONIC PAIN ASSESSMENT

DATE		DAY	
TIME STARTED		TIME ENDED	
TOTAL DURATION			

RIGHT SIDE   BACK   FRONT   LEFT SIDE

LEFT   RIGHT   RIGHT   LEFT

Mark the location of the pain

LENGTH OF TIME EXPERIENCING THE PAIN?

< 6 Months		6-12 Months
1-3 Years		3 Years +

TYPE OF PAIN

Indescribable	Stabbing	Sharp
Burning	Aching	Prickly
Numb	Tingling/ Pins & Needles	
Other		

EXTERNAL ENVIROMENTAL FACTORS

Sun/ Heat	Cold	Windy
Rain	Aching	Cloudy
Other		

PAIN SCALE

NO PAIN ———————————————→ SEVERE PAIN

0	1	2	3	4	5	6	7	8	9	10

SUSPECTED TRIGGERS

-
-
-
-

-
-
-
-

SYMPTOMS

RELIEF MEASURES

NOTES

CHRONIC PAIN ASSESSMENT

DATE		DAY	
TIME STARTED		TIME ENDED	
TOTAL DURATION			

RIGHT SIDE　　BACK　　FRONT　　LEFT SIDE

LEFT　RIGHT　RIGHT　LEFT

← ────────── Mark the location of the pain

LENGTH OF TIME EXPERIENCING THE PAIN?

< 6 Months		6-12 Months
1-3 Years		3 Years +

TYPE OF PAIN

Indescribable	Stabbing	Sharp
Burning	Aching	Prickly
Numb	Tingling/ Pins & Needles	
Other		

EXTERNAL ENVIROMENTAL FACTORS

Sun/ Heat	Cold	Windy
Rain	Aching	Cloudy
Other		

PAIN SCALE

NO PAIN ──────────────────────→ SEVERE PAIN

0	1	2	3	4	5	6	7	8	9	10

SUSPECTED TRIGGERS

- _____
- _____
- _____
- _____

- _____
- _____
- _____
- _____

SYMPTOMS

RELIEF MEASURES

NOTES

CHRONIC PAIN ASSESSMENT

DATE		DAY	
TIME STARTED		TIME ENDED	
TOTAL DURATION			

RIGHT SIDE   BACK   FRONT   LEFT SIDE

← Mark the location of the pain

LENGTH OF TIME EXPERIENCING THE PAIN?

< 6 Months		6-12 Months	
1-3 Years		3 Years +	

TYPE OF PAIN

Indescribable		Stabbing		Sharp	
Burning		Aching		Prickly	
Numb		Tingling/ Pins & Needles			
Other					

EXTERNAL ENVIROMENTAL FACTORS

Sun/ Heat		Cold		Windy	
Rain		Aching		Cloudy	
Other					

PAIN SCALE

NO PAIN ————————————————————→ SEVERE PAIN

0	1	2	3	4	5	6	7	8	9	10

SUSPECTED TRIGGERS

-
-
-
-

-
-
-
-

SYMPTOMS

RELIEF MEASURES

NOTES

CHRONIC PAIN ASSESSMENT

DATE		DAY	
TIME STARTED		TIME ENDED	
TOTAL DURATION			

RIGHT SIDE   BACK   FRONT   LEFT SIDE

LEFT   RIGHT   RIGHT   LEFT

← Mark the location of the pain

LENGTH OF TIME EXPERIENCING THE PAIN?

< 6 Months		6-12 Months	
1-3 Years		3 Years +	

TYPE OF PAIN

Indescribable		Stabbing		Sharp	
Burning		Aching		Prickly	
Numb		Tingling/ Pins & Needles			
Other					

EXTERNAL ENVIROMENTAL FACTORS

Sun/ Heat		Cold		Windy	
Rain		Aching		Cloudy	
Other					

PAIN SCALE

NO PAIN ————————————————→ SEVERE PAIN

0	1	2	3	4	5	6	7	8	9	10

SUSPECTED TRIGGERS

-
-
-
-

-
-
-
-

SYMPTOMS

RELIEF MEASURES

NOTES

TREATMENT HISTORY- PRESCRIPTION MEDICATION

MEDICATION NAME	DATE STARTED	START DOSE	DATE ENDED	END DOSE

RESULT & NOTES	

MEDICATION NAME	DATE STARTED	START DOSE	DATE ENDED	END DOSE

RESULT & NOTES	

MEDICATION NAME	DATE STARTED	START DOSE	DATE ENDED	END DOSE

RESULT & NOTES	

MEDICATION NAME	DATE STARTED	START DOSE	DATE ENDED	END DOSE

RESULT & NOTES	

MEDICATION NAME	DATE STARTED	START DOSE	DATE ENDED	END DOSE

RESULT & NOTES	

MEDICATION NAME	DATE STARTED	START DOSE	DATE ENDED	END DOSE

RESULT & NOTES	

MEDICATION NAME	DATE STARTED	START DOSE	DATE ENDED	END DOSE

RESULT & NOTES	

TREATMENT HISTORY- NON PRESCRIPTION

DESCRIPTION	DATE	RESULTS & NOTES

DESCRIPTION	DATE	RESULTS & NOTES

DESCRIPTION	DATE	RESULTS & NOTES

DESCRIPTION	DATE	RESULTS & NOTES

DESCRIPTION	DATE	RESULTS & NOTES

DESCRIPTION	DATE	RESULTS & NOTES

DESCRIPTION	DATE	RESULTS & NOTES

DESCRIPTION	DATE	RESULTS & NOTES

DESCRIPTION	DATE	RESULTS & NOTES

DESCRIPTION	DATE	RESULTS & NOTES

DESCRIPTION	DATE	RESULTS & NOTES

DESCRIPTION	DATE	RESULTS & NOTES

DESCRIPTION	DATE	RESULTS & NOTES

TREATMENT HISTORY- PRESCRIPTION MEDICATION

MEDICATION NAME	DATE STARTED	START DOSE	DATE ENDED	END DOSE

RESULT & NOTES	

MEDICATION NAME	DATE STARTED	START DOSE	DATE ENDED	END DOSE

RESULT & NOTES	

MEDICATION NAME	DATE STARTED	START DOSE	DATE ENDED	END DOSE

RESULT & NOTES	

MEDICATION NAME	DATE STARTED	START DOSE	DATE ENDED	END DOSE

RESULT & NOTES	

MEDICATION NAME	DATE STARTED	START DOSE	DATE ENDED	END DOSE

RESULT & NOTES	

MEDICATION NAME	DATE STARTED	START DOSE	DATE ENDED	END DOSE

RESULT & NOTES	

MEDICATION NAME	DATE STARTED	START DOSE	DATE ENDED	END DOSE

RESULT & NOTES	

TREATMENT HISTORY- NON PRESCRIPTION

DESCRIPTION	DATE	RESULTS & NOTES

DESCRIPTION	DATE	RESULTS & NOTES

DESCRIPTION	DATE	RESULTS & NOTES

DESCRIPTION	DATE	RESULTS & NOTES

DESCRIPTION	DATE	RESULTS & NOTES

DESCRIPTION	DATE	RESULTS & NOTES

DESCRIPTION	DATE	RESULTS & NOTES

DESCRIPTION	DATE	RESULTS & NOTES

DESCRIPTION	DATE	RESULTS & NOTES

DESCRIPTION	DATE	RESULTS & NOTES

DESCRIPTION	DATE	RESULTS & NOTES

DESCRIPTION	DATE	RESULTS & NOTES

DESCRIPTION	DATE	RESULTS & NOTES

DESCRIPTION	DATE	RESULTS & NOTES

DOCTORS/ CLINIC APPOINTMENTS

DATE	TIME	WITH	REASON

NOTES/ RESULT

_____
_____
_____

DATE	TIME	WITH	REASON

NOTES/ RESULT

_____
_____
_____

DATE	TIME	WITH	REASON

NOTES/ RESULT

_____
_____
_____

DATE	TIME	WITH	REASON

NOTES/ RESULT

_____
_____
_____

DATE	TIME	WITH	REASON

NOTES/ RESULT

_____
_____
_____

DATE	TIME	WITH	REASON
NOTES/ RESULT			

_____

_____

_____

_____

DATE	TIME	WITH	REASON
NOTES/ RESULT			

_____

_____

_____

_____

DATE	TIME	WITH	REASON
NOTES/ RESULT			

_____

_____

_____

_____

DATE	TIME	WITH	REASON
NOTES/ RESULT			

_____

_____

_____

_____

DATE	TIME	WITH	REASON
NOTES/ RESULT			

_____

_____

_____

_____

DOCTORS/ CLINIC APPOINTMENTS

DATE	TIME	WITH	REASON
NOTES/ RESULT			

_____
_____
_____

DATE	TIME	WITH	REASON
NOTES/ RESULT			

_____
_____
_____

DATE	TIME	WITH	REASON
NOTES/ RESULT			

_____
_____
_____

DATE	TIME	WITH	REASON
NOTES/ RESULT			

_____
_____
_____

DATE	TIME	WITH	REASON
NOTES/ RESULT			

_____
_____
_____

DATE	TIME	WITH	REASON

NOTES/ RESULT

DATE	TIME	WITH	REASON

NOTES/ RESULT

DATE	TIME	WITH	REASON

NOTES/ RESULT

DATE	TIME	WITH	REASON

NOTES/ RESULT

DATE	TIME	WITH	REASON

NOTES/ RESULT

DOCTORS/ CLINIC APPOINTMENTS

DATE	TIME	WITH	REASON
NOTES/ RESULT			

DATE	TIME	WITH	REASON
NOTES/ RESULT			

DATE	TIME	WITH	REASON
NOTES/ RESULT			

DATE	TIME	WITH	REASON
NOTES/ RESULT			

DATE	TIME	WITH	REASON
NOTES/ RESULT			

DATE	TIME	WITH	REASON
NOTES/ RESULT			

DATE	TIME	WITH	REASON
NOTES/ RESULT			

DATE	TIME	WITH	REASON
NOTES/ RESULT			

DATE	TIME	WITH	REASON
NOTES/ RESULT			

DATE	TIME	WITH	REASON
NOTES/ RESULT			

NOTES

Made in the USA
Columbia, SC
13 November 2019